Management of Chemotherapy-Induced Nausea and Vomiting

Rudolph M. Navari
Editor

Management of Chemotherapy-Induced Nausea and Vomiting

New Agents and New Uses of Current Agents

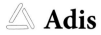 Adis

Editor
Rudolph M. Navari
Medicine
Indiana University School of Medicine
South Bend
Indiana
USA

ISBN 978-3-319-27014-2   ISBN 978-3-319-27016-6   (eBook)
DOI 10.1007/978-3-319-27016-6

Library of Congress Control Number: 2016930399

Springer Cham Heidelberg New York Dordrecht London

Printed on acid-free paper

Adis is a brand of Springer
Springer International Publishing AG Switzerland is part of Springer Science+Business Media
(www.springer.com)

Biography

Rudolph M. Navari, M.D., Ph.D., F.A.C.P.
Director, Cancer Care Program, Central and South America
World Health Organization
Professor of Medicine
Indiana University School of Medicine South Bend
Medical Director, Student Outreach Clinic
Indiana University School of Medicine South Bend

Dr. Navari received the Ph.D. degree at the University of Virginia and the M.D. degree at the Medical College of Virginia. He received training in internal medicine at the University of Alabama in Birmingham and was a fellow in hematology and oncology at the Fred Hutchinson Cancer Research Center, University of Washington School of Medicine. He is board certified in internal medicine and medical oncology. From 1983 to 1998, he served on the Clinical Faculty of the University of Alabama Birmingham and was a practicing medical oncologist in the Simon-Williamson Clinic. During this time, he was chairman of the Department of Medicine and president of the Simon-Williamson Clinic, director of the Bone Marrow Transplantation Program, and director of the Comprehensive Cancer Program at Baptist Medical Center. In 1997, he was elected a fellow of the American College of Physicians. During 1998–1999, he was a fellow in clinical medical ethics in the MacLean Center for Clinical Medical Ethics at the University of Chicago. He joined the faculty of the College of Science of the University of Notre Dame (UND) in 1999 as director of the Walther Cancer Research Center. He was appointed associate dean, College of Science, in 2000. In July, 2005, he became professor of medicine, assistant dean, and director, Indiana University School of Medicine South Bend (IUSM SB), and adjunct professor of biochemistry, University of Notre Dame. In 2011, he was appointed clinical director, Harper Cancer Research Institute, a partnership between IUSM SB and UND. He was promoted to associate dean in 2012. Along with the medical students at IUSM SB, he founded the IUSM SB Student Outreach Clinic in 2013 and was appointed the Clinic's first medical director.

In 2014, he joined the World Health Organization as director of the Cancer Care Program, Eastern Europe. In 2015, he was appointed director of the Cancer Care Program, Central and South America.

Dr. Navari's research interests include supportive care in clinical oncology, development of antiemetics, palliative care, and the doctor-patient relationship in clinical oncology. He has published over 130 peer-reviewed articles, with the most recent dealing with supportive care issues in clinical oncology

Contents

Chapter 1
Introduction

Rudolph M. Navari

Chemotherapy-induced nausea and vomiting (CINV) is associated with a significant deterioration in quality of life and is perceived by patients as a major adverse effect of the treatment [1, 2]. Increased risk of CINV is associated with the type of chemotherapy administered (Table 1.1) and specific patient characteristics (Table 1.2) [3]. CINV can result in serious complications, such as weakness, weight loss, electrolyte imbalance, dehydration, or anorexia, and is associated with a variety of complications, including fractures, esophageal tears, decline in behavioral and mental status, and wound dehiscence [1]. Patients who are dehydrated, debilitated, or malnourished, as well as those who have an electrolyte imbalance or those who have recently undergone surgery or radiation therapy, are at greater risk of experiencing serious complications from CINV [1–3].

The use of 5-hydroxytryptamine-3 (5-HT$_3$) receptor antagonists plus dexamethasone has improved the control of CINV [4]. Recent studies have demonstrated some improvement in the control of CINV with the use of a number of new agents: palonosetron, a second-generation 5-HT$_3$ receptor antagonist [4]; neurokinin (NK)$_1$ receptor antagonists aprepitant [5, 6], netupitant [7], and rolapitant [8]; and olanzapine, an antipsychotic that blocks multiple neurotransmitters in the central nervous system [9–11].

The primary end point used for studies evaluating various agents for the control of CINV has been complete response (no emesis, no use of rescue medication) over the acute (24 h post-chemotherapy), delayed (24–120 h), and overall (0–120 h) periods [3]. Recent studies have shown that the combination of a 5-HT$_3$ receptor antagonist, dexamethasone, and an NK$_1$ receptor antagonist have improved the control of emesis in patients receiving either highly emetogenic chemotherapy (HEC)

R.M. Navari, MD, PhD, FACP
Cancer Care Program, Central and South America, World Health Organization, Indiana University School of Medicine South Bend, South Bend, IN, USA
e-mail: rmnavari@gmail.com

© Springer International Publishing Switzerland 2016
R.M. Navari (ed.), *Management of Chemotherapy-Induced Nausea and Vomiting: New Agents and New Uses of Current Agents*,
DOI 10.1007/978-3-319-27016-6_1

1

Table 1.1 Emetic potential of chemotherapy agents

Emetogenic potential	Typical agents	Definition (no CINV prevention)
High	Cisplatin, dacarbazine, melphalan (high dose), nitrogen mustard, cyclophosphamide plus an anthracycline	Emesis in nearly all patients
Moderate	Anthracyclines, carboplatin, carmustine (high dose), cyclophosphamide, ifosfamide, irinotecan, methotrexate (high dose), oxaliplatin, topotecan	Emesis in >70 % of patients
Low	Etoposide, 5-fluorouracil, gemcitabine, mitoxantrone, taxanes, vinblastine, vinorelbine	Emesis in 10–70 % of patients
Minimal	Bortezomib, hormones, vinca alkaloids, bleomycin	Emesis in <10 % of patients

CINV chemotherapy-induced nausea and vomiting

Table 1.2 Patient-related risk factors for emesis following chemotherapy

Major factors	Minor factors
Female, age <50 years, history of low prior chronic alcohol intake (<1 oz of alcohol/day), history of previous chemotherapy-induced emesis	History of motion sickness, emesis during past pregnancy

or moderately emetogenic chemotherapy (MEC) over a 120-h period following chemotherapy administration [5, 6]. Many of these same studies have measured nausea as a secondary end point and have demonstrated that nausea has not been well controlled [12].

Emesis is a well-defined event that is easily measured, but nausea may be more subjective and more difficult to measure. However, two well-defined measures of nausea that appear to be effective and reproducible measurement tools are the visual analogue scale (VAS) and the Likert scale [13]. The VAS is a scale from 0 to 10 or 0 to 100, with zero representing no nausea and 10 or 100 representing maximal nausea. The Likert scale asks patients to rate nausea as "none, mild, moderate, or severe."

Many studies have reported the secondary end point of "no significant nausea" or "only mild nausea" [3–6]. Studies that have reported "no nausea" may be more useful in identifying the most effective available anti-nausea agents [12].

Despite the introduction of more effective antiemetic agents, emesis and nausea remain a significant complication of chemotherapy. The purpose of this text is to evaluate the clinical agents available for the prevention and treatment of CINV. The use of these agents in various clinical settings is described using the recently established guidelines from the Multinational Association of Supportive Care in Cancer (MASCC) and the European Society of Medical Oncology (ESMO) [14], the American Society of Clinical Oncology (ASCO) [15], and the National Comprehensive Cancer Network (NCCN) guidelines [16]. The literature cited in the text consists of the primary clinical trials used for the US FDA approval of the various agents as well as recent comprehensive reviews.

References

1. Bloechl-Daum B, Deuson RR, Mavros P et al (2006) Delayed nausea and vomiting continue to reduce patients' quality of life after highly and moderately emetogenic chemotherapy despite antiemetic treatment. J Clin Oncol 24:4472–4478
2. Cohen L, de Moor CA, Eisenberg P et al (2007) Chemotherapy-induced nausea and vomiting: incidence and impact on patient quality of life at community oncology settings. Support Care Cancer 15(5):497–503
3. Navari RM (2009) Pharmacological management of chemotherapy-induced nausea and vomiting: focus on recent developments. Drugs 69:515–533
4. Navari RM (2010) Palonosetron for the prevention of chemotherapy-induced nausea and vomiting in patients with cancer. Future Oncol 6:1074–1084
5. Curran MP, Robinson DM (2009) Aprepitant: a review of its use in the prevention of nausea and vomiting. Drugs 69:1853–1858
6. Sankhala KK, Pandya DM, Sarantopoulos J et al (2009) Prevention of chemotherapy induced nausea and vomiting: a focus on aprepitant. Expert Opin Drug Metab Toxicol 12:1607–1614
7. Navari RM (2015) Profile of netupitant/palonosetron fixed dose combination (NEPA) and its potential in the treatment of chemotherapy-induced nausea and vomiting (CINV). Drug Des Dev Ther 9:155–161
8. Navari RM (2015) Rolapitant for the treatment of chemotherapy induced nausea and vomiting. Expert Rev Anticancer Ther 15:1127–1133
9. Navari RM, Einhorn LH, Loehrer PJ et al (2007) A phase II trial of olanzapine, dexamethasone, and palonosetron for the prevention of chemotherapy-induced nausea and vomiting. Support Care Cancer 15:1285–1291
10. Tan L, Liu J, Liu X et al (2009) Clinical research of olanzapine for the prevention of chemotherapy-induced nausea and vomiting. J Exp Clin Cancer Res 28:1–7
11. Navari RM, Gray SE, Kerr AC (2011) Olanzapine versus aprepitant for the prevention of chemotherapy-induced nausea and vomiting: a randomized phase III trial. J Support Oncol 9:188–195
12. Navari RM (2012) Treatment of chemotherapy-induced nausea. Community Oncol 9:20–26
13. Stern RM, Koch KL, Andrews PLR (eds) (2011) Nausea: mechanisms and management. Oxford University Press, New York
14. Roila F, Herrstedt J, Aapro M et al (2010) Guideline update for MASCC and ESMO in the prevention of chemotherapy- and radiotherapy-induced nausea and vomiting: results of the Perugia consensus conference. Ann Oncol 21(5):232–243
15. Basch E, Prestrud AA, Hesketh PJ et al (2011) Antiemetic American Society Clinical Oncology clinical practice guideline update. J Clin Oncol 29:4189–4198
16. NCCN Clinical Practice Guidelines in Oncology version 1 2015. Antiemesis. National Comprehensive Cancer Network (NCCN) [online]. Available from URL: http://www.nccn.org/professionals/physician_gls/PDF/antiemesis.pdf. Accessed Oct 2015

Chapter 2
The Physiology and Pharmacology of Nausea and Vomiting Induced by Anticancer Chemotherapy in Humans

Paul L.R. Andrews and John A. Rudd

2.1 Introduction

It is approximately 100 years since the fortuitous observation of lymphoid aplasia in soldiers exposed to the chemical warfare agent mustard gas led to the therapeutic use of nitrogen mustard in 1946 for Hodgkin's lymphoma [17, 65]. However, nitrogen mustard also induced emesis revealing the unfortunate link between diverse treatments for cancer and their ability to induce emesis, a pattern which continued with the introduction of radiotherapy and other chemotherapeutic agents (cyclophosphamide and 5-fluorouracil) and which was brought into particular focus by the introduction of cisplatin in the 1970s [26]. The profound and protracted nausea and vomiting provoked by cisplatin acted as a stimulus to preclinical research to understand the mechanism(s) and pathway(s) by which chemotherapeutic agents induced emesis and to identify more effective anti-emetic agents that were available at the time (e.g. belladonna-scopolamine family, metoclopramide, nabilone, prochlorperazine; see [5], 2014 for refs.). These studies led to the identification of the anti-emetic effect of 5-hydroxytryptamine$_3$ (5-HT$_3$) receptor antagonists which was recognised in the "top five" advances in oncology in the last 50 years (http://www.asco.org/advocacy/votes-are-top-5-advances-50-years-modern-oncology) further emphasising the significance of this side effect for patients. Subsequently the involvement of substance P and neurokinin$_1$ (NK$_1$) receptors in emesis was identified (see [8] for review) giving rise to the anti-emetic combination of a 5-HT$_3$ and NK$_1$ receptor antagonist (e.g. NEPA (netupitant+palonosetron)), [72].

P.L.R. Andrews, DSc (✉)
Division of Biomedical Sciences, St George's University of London, London, UK
e-mail: pandrews@sgul.ac.uk

J.A. Rudd, PhD
School of Biomedical Sciences, and Brain and Mind Institute, The Chinese University of Hong Kong, Shatin, New Territories, Hong Kong, SAR, China

© Springer International Publishing Switzerland 2016
R.M. Navari (ed.), *Management of Chemotherapy-Induced Nausea and Vomiting: New Agents and New Uses of Current Agents*,
DOI 10.1007/978-3-319-27016-6_2

This chapter reviews the general and specific mechanisms underlying the induction of chemotherapy-induced nausea and vomiting (CINV).

2.2   Why Should Anticancer Therapies Induce Nausea and Vomiting? An Evolutionary Perspective

Nausea and vomiting are considered to be part of the mechanisms by which the body defends itself against toxins accidentally ingested with the food. Some of these toxins are from plants (e.g. lycorine from daffodils; digoxin from foxglove; vinca alkaloids from periwinkle; morphine from the opium poppy) and paradoxically include chemicals used therapeutically, fungi (e.g. vomitoxin and other trichothecenes) and algae (e.g. brevetoxin), whilst others are of bacterial (e.g. Staphylococcal enterotoxin), viral (e.g. norovirus, rotavirus) or animal (e.g. physaelamin, tetrodotox) in origin. Broadly speaking, nausea acts as a warning so that further intake is reduced and gastric emptying is delayed to confine potentially contaminated food to the stomach from where it is expelled by vomiting [35]. Nausea also leads to a learned aversion causing avoidance of that food in the future. Even the evolution of motion sickness can be viewed within this "toxin detection model" [119, 123, 164]. Clearly in the natural world such responses to an ingested toxin have survival value, but in the context of the clinic when triggered by a disease treatment, the same response is perceived as drug "side effects" or "adverse events". In the case of ingested toxins, gastric acid and digestive enzymes may degrade some toxins, whilst the vomiting can void any toxin that is confined to the upper gut. However, in the case of intravenous anticancer chemotherapy, the "the toxin" (i.e. the drug) is in the circulation, and vomiting will have no effect upon the levels so the response is likely to be protracted until metabolism or excretion intervenes; this is analogous to the situation when vomiting follows a venomous bite where the toxin is also in the circulation. Additionally, learning to avoid a food associated with previous illness is important for survival, but aversion to, and subsequent avoidance of, a therapy leads to suboptimal treatment but such a learned aversion provides a model within which to understand (and potentially treat) anticipatory nausea and vomiting (see below).

Why should agents with a diverse range of chemical structures targeted at a wide range of different molecular targets in cancer cells trigger nausea and vomiting as adverse events? The simple answer is that the anticancer agent via one or more of its chemical properties is able to activate one or more of the pathways (see below) which evolved to deal with natural toxins ingested with the food. It should be noted that some of the anticancer agents are derived from naturally occurring plant toxins. The non-cancerous cells in patients with cancer are known to be variably affected by anticancer drugs, and the "cells" involved in induction of emesis could be regarded as part of these off-target effects of chemotherapy agents.

Whist we have drugs (anti-emetics) that can affect nausea and vomiting induced by chemotherapeutic agents to varying degrees, this means that we understand the pharmacology of the evolved emetic pathways, but it does not mean that we understand exactly *how* chemotherapy agents activate the pathways. If we understood what properties the chemotherapeutic agents have in common which leads to the activation of emetic pathways, it may be possible to design agents devoid of emetic liability provided that the anticancer and emetogenic properties do not have the same molecular mechanism(s).

2.3 Animal Models vs. the Clinic and the Problems of Studying Nausea in Humans

2.3.1 Cancer Patients and Animal Models: Limitations

Although there are examples of classes of anti-emetic that have their origins in traditional remedies (e.g. ginger, scopolamine [henbane]), in popular culture (cannabis smoking) and from pursuit of anecdotal reports of emesis being reduced by a drug used to treat an indication not associated with emesis (e.g. H_1 antagonist being used to treat urticaria affecting car sickness; see [5]), the newer anti-emetics (5-HT$_3$ and NK$_1$ receptor antagonists) have come from fundamental studies of the neuropharmacology of emesis in animals. The utility of the animal models relies on their ability to translate to a human patient, and this in turn relies on the overall response reflecting the pattern of the human response (e.g. acute and delayed phase), the pathway(s) activated by the emetic challenge (e.g. cisplatin) being the same as in the patient and that the various molecular mechanisms (e.g. transmitter/receptors) at which the drug is targeted are also the same. For emetic challenges such as motion, the dopamine receptor agonist apomorphine acting on the area postrema, and the gastric irritant ipecacuanha, it is possible to investigate the anti-emetic efficacy of a candidate in healthy volunteers assuming it has passed safety toxicology. However, such human models may not reflect the mechanisms operating during chemotherapy and have to be interpreted with caution as, for example, whilst motion-induced emesis is unaffected by the 5-hydroxytryptamine$_3$ receptor antagonist ondansetron, ipecacuanha-induced emesis is reduced or abolished [54, 153].

A range of animal species have been used particularly over the last 30 years to investigate the pharmacology of the emetic response to cytotoxic drugs although cisplatin has most frequently been used as it is perceived as the most potent challenge. The ferret has been the species subject to the most detailed investigation and has become the standard model for testing anti-emetic efficacy of novel chemical entities and was the species in which the initial anti-emetic effect of both 5-HT$_3$ and NK$_1$ receptor antagonists was first identified (for review see Percie du Sert and Andrews [125]). Other species in which cisplatin induces an emetic response include cat [142], dog [128], house musk shrew (*Suncus murinus*; [167]), least shrew (*Cryptotis parva*; [33]) and pigeon [168]. Although rats and other rodents do not vomit [79], they have also been used to investigate the effects of cisplatin by monitoring pica (kaolin consumption; [159]), conditioned taste aversion [141], vagal afferent activity [80], nerve transection [36] and brain c-Fos activity [37, 78].

A detailed discussion of the limitations of the various animal species used to identify potential anti-emetic agents is beyond the scope of this review, but in each case it must be borne in mind that the animal studies are investigating cisplatin-induced emesis and are not attempting to mimic chemotherapy in a cancer patient. Much of the mechanistic evidence comes from animal studies of single agents, but it is now rare to use single-agent chemotherapy, and this emphasises that the animal studies are not attempting to mimic chemotherapy. Apart from any fundamental animal vs. human differences in emetic pathways and pharmacology, the differences between the effects of a single emetic chemotherapeutic substance in a healthy animal and a patient with cancer being treated with chemotherapy and concomitant medication help to account for some differences in efficacy. Looking broadly at anti-emetics investigated in the ferret against cisplatin when the same compounds have been investigated in patients, the agents have all had some efficacy, but the magnitude of the effects against vomiting has often differed, with the compounds usually being more effective in the animal (see [126]). Comparing efficacy of anti-emetics between animal studies and patients is difficult because apart from the problems of assessing nausea discussed below, the level of detail collected about number of retches and vomits and their timing is much greater in the animals than in humans, so direct comparison of efficacy measures is problematic.

Our understanding of the physiology of the sensation of nausea is rudimentary in contrast to that of the mechanics of vomiting and its central control. Researching nausea is problematic, and some of the constraints are outlined briefly below to provide background to the subsequent section on the physiology.

2.3.2   The Problems of Studying Nausea in Humans

2.3.2.1   Definition

Nausea is a self-reported sensation that is remarkably difficult to define precisely (see [154] for 30 definitions), but an analysis of definitions shows the common key features: (a) it is *unpleasant* but is clearly different from pain; (b) the sensation is frequently, but not always, *associated with the stomach*, but this does not mean that this is the site of origin as the sensation could be referred; (c) it is *aversive* and can lead to avoidance of an associated cause; (d) it is associated with a *desire to vomit or the feeling that vomiting is imminent* but is not necessarily accompanied by vomiting and can continue even after vomiting has occurred often following a brief period of relief; and (e) it can *occur in waves*, waxing and waning although the periodicity has never been measured. Visual analogue or self-report scales rely on providing a definition of nausea which, it is hoped, overlaps with some aspect of the patient's experience or understanding or requires the patient to self-define nausea which assumes that in a particular study all patients are reporting the same phenomenon. Scoring is usually completed retrospectively so relies on recall at a time when patients may be distressed; additionally it is not ideal to ask patients to complete the measurement tool at multiple time points as this could itself trigger thoughts of nausea, but the consequence is that the data on the temporal sequence of nausea is poor. The meaning of scores using VAS and the ways in which they are categorised into categories like "no significant nausea" to assess changes in anti-emetic trials is also a cause for concern [5]. Many of these problems could be overcome by using biomarkers, but as described in the section below, this is also problematic.

2.3.2.2 Biomarkers

Although peer assessment has been used with some success by navy sailors as a method to assess the physical symptoms and performance impact of seasickness [63], such methods are not easily applied to the clinic where nausea and vomiting are the specific symptoms of interest. Additionally in studies where the patient's and the clinician's assessment of symptoms has been compared, the clinician typically underestimates the severity in comparison to the patient [40]. A method of identifying the occurrence and magnitude of nausea in real time, independent of the need for self-reporting by the patient, would enable more objective measurement and characterisation of the time course of nausea and of the impact of anti-emetics. In addition, it would be possible to measure nausea in situations where reporting is problematic such as in neonates and babies and in stroke patients [5]. Potential approaches are based upon measurement of the physiological changes which accompany nausea and which are described below.

2.3.2.3 Investigating Nausea in Patients and Healthy Volunteers

The frequent occurrence of nausea in patients should make researching the underlying mechanisms relatively simple, but there are both ethical and practical constraints. Studies in patients undergoing chemotherapy have predominantly involved measurement of substances in the plasma and attempted correlation with nausea or vomiting. Such studies whilst providing a useful description of the events occurring in a patient have a limited temporal resolution and may be difficult to interpret because patient populations are not homogeneous with confounding factors (co-morbidity, multiple medications). We are aware of only one study of brain imaging (see below) investigating nausea in patients undergoing chemotherapy [56]. The majority of knowledge of the physiology of nausea comes from studies of healthy (usually young) volunteers using illusory self-motion (vection) as a stimulus. Although vection has the advantage that the volunteer can terminate the study by closing their eyes, the question arises about how representative visually induced motion sickness is of nausea induced either by "real" motion or pharmacological challenges (e.g. apomorphine, ipecacuanha) in healthy volunteers or chemotherapy in cancer patients [154]. Currently there is no evidence that the sensation of nausea evoked by the various stimuli differs, although the descriptions of the sensation being variously associated with the stomach, throat or head make this a possibility. Studies using fMRI in healthy volunteers experiencing nausea have begun to identify regions concerned with the sensation and accompanying autonomic changes, but again these are limited to vection as a stimulus. It is to be hoped that the introduction of more open design types of scanner will permit studies in patients. Considerable advances have been made in the production of radioligands suitable for use in humans so it should soon be possible to identify the transmitters/receptors in the brain areas implicated in nausea by brain imaging which is described below [49, 120, 121, 146].

2.3.2.4   Assessing Efficacy of Anti-emetics Against Nausea

There are clearly practical considerations in the methodology that can be used in clinical trials to assess nausea and vomiting, but it is important to be aware of methodological problems that make it difficult to define exactly what the drug is doing. It often said that vomiting is more affected or better treated than nausea by anti-emetics, but it is difficult to find robust data to enable an assessment of the extent of this difference for different anti-emetic agents [5]. Comparing efficacy against nausea as compared to vomiting is difficult unless both are totally blocked as the comparison relies on comparing data derived from a VAS/self-report scale vs. data on number of emetic episodes (comprised of retches and vomits). What do changes in the VAS score actually mean in terms of the relationship to either the intensity of the stimulus or pathway activation? For many sensory experiences, the stimulus is related to the sensory experience by a log-power relationship, but we do not know the relationship for the induction of nausea. A study of motion sickness showed that the reported gastrointestinal sensations increased disproportionately with time in the rotating chair [117]. Although scoring emesis appears more precise because "episodes" are often used, it is possible to have a reduction in total number of retches and vomits that would not be reflected in the score if an episode is made up of more than one bout of retching and vomiting. In addition, if retrospective recall of number of episodes is used (assuming the anti-emetic drug has no amnesic properties!), this further adds inaccuracies and incidentally can make direct comparison of preclinical and clinical data difficult in the context of assessing translation of animal models to the clinic. The impact of reducing emesis upon the nausea score is rarely considered.

2.3.2.5   Can Nausea Be Studied in Animals?

Sensu stricto the answer to this question is clearly "no" as it is a self-reported sensation and hence requires the ability to identify, classify and communicate (usually verbally). This comment does not deny that in response to an emetic stimulus animals have a sensory experience with at least functional equivalence to the sensation of nausea reported by humans and this is well demonstrated by the genesis of learned food aversions and avoidance in multiple species [5, 154]. Many studies of "nausea" have been performed in rodents as they lack the ability to vomit because of differences in the anatomy of the digestive tract and diaphragm and organisation of the brainstem [79], but this also begs the question of what other differences may exist in their brain organisation. Studies in animals aimed at providing insights into nausea have used a variety of measurements including conditioned taste aversion/ avoidance, pica (kaolin consumption), conditioned gaping and quantification of a range of behaviours occurring in the peri-emesis period (e.g. licking, chin rubbing, digging) (for refs. see [154], Chap. 8). More recently brain neuronal activation in response to emetic stimuli has been studied using c-Fos immunohistochemistry and has identified activation of "higher" brain regions (e.g. insular cortex, central nucleus of the amygdala), and such studies may provide insights into potential drug targets, but they need to be considered with caution in view of differences in brain anatomy and likely differences in transmitter and receptor systems from humans. In addition, c-Fos only shows neurones that are active (after at least 30 min stimulation), whereas in volunteers experiencing nausea brain imaging has demonstrated areas of the brain with decreased as well as increased activity [49].

2.4 The Physiology of Nausea

Bearing the above constraints in mind, we will summarise what is known of the physiological changes that accompany nausea and the way in which the sensation itself is generated in humans, but data from some animal studies will be used to illustrate additional points. For simplicity we will separate the endocrine, autonomic and brain changes, but understanding the temporal sequence is critical to understanding how the sensation is produced. In principle there are three working models for the genesis of the sensation and they are not mutually exclusive:

1. Stimulation of the input pathways (area postrema, vestibular system, abdominal vagal afferents) at a level above that involved in homeostatic functions (e.g. balance, regulation of food intake, vago-vagal motility reflexes) but below that required to evoke vomiting activates a pathway within the brain leading to genesis of the sensation of nausea via activation of specific cortical nuclei. Conceptually this is the least complex mechanism and readily explains how nausea can be evoked by motion stimuli, drugs acting on the area postrema (apomorphine) and vagal afferent activation (disordered gastric motility, acute cisplatin emesis) without the intervention of any intermediate processes.

2. Stimulation of the input pathways at a level above that involved in homeostatic functions but below that required to evoke vomiting causes modulation of autonomic outflows to disrupt gastric myoelectric activity (GMA), and this provides the signal for nausea via visceral afferents and then brain pathways. However,

GMA can be disrupted without induction of nausea (e.g. feeding) so unless the pattern is very specific, this mechanism operating *alone* appears unlikely.

3. Stimulation of the input pathways at a level above that involved in homeostatic functions but below that required to evoke vomiting causes a secretion of "high concentration" of vasopressin (oxytocin in the rodents) which either evokes nausea directly by accessing central pathways via the CVOs (most likely AP) or disrupts the GMA which is then detected and signalled to the brain as described above.

Deciding between these options relies on studies with a high temporal resolution but also a knowledge of the magnitude of changes in the GMA and AVP required for nausea to be reported. The above options are not mutually exclusive as nausea can still occur in the absence of changes in plasma AVP (e.g. diabetes insipidus, mild vection) and patients with total gastrectomy or high spinal cord lesions. Understanding which effects are primary and which are secondary is important for identifying targets for antinausea drugs; for example, vasopressin receptor antagonists would be effective in #3 but not #1 or #2.

Below we summarise the changes in hormones, the autonomic nervous system and the brain that have been described in subjects reporting nausea and focus on the issues of the magnitude of the response, its temporal relationship to reports of nausea and whether the changes seen provide a plausible mechanism for genesis of the sensation. The reader is referred to the book by Stern and colleagues [154] for detailed discussions and additional references [154].

2.4.1 Hormones

The hormone most extensively studied and consistently (but not universally) linked to nausea is vasopressin (AVP, antidiuretic hormone (ADH)) synthesised in the supraoptic and paraventricular nuclei and secreted into the blood stream from the posterior pituitary. AVP, but not oxytocin, has been shown to increase in the plasma in humans following apomorphine [50, 122, 137], cholecystokinin [102], motion and vection [46, 49, 178] and anticancer chemotherapy [13, 42, 53]. Several studies reported that the nausea score positively correlated (often not a strong correlation) with [AVP] or that nausea was only present in subjects with a significant change in [AVP]. The magnitude of the plasma [AVP] changes is highly variable across the studies and is not obviously related to the stimulus; changes range from ~5× to ~500×. The temporal resolution of plasma AVP measurement is relatively poor so the exact temporal relationship between symptoms and [AVP] is not well defined, but in general plasma AVP rises in concert with the reports of nausea and in the few cases where vomiting ensued the rise in AVP occurred prior to vomiting. Systemic administration of AVP in humans is capable of inducing nausea [24, 89] and vomiting [160] with nausea (and abdominal cramping) occurring within 5 min of the start of the infusion [24]. There are no publications of the effects of selective vasopressin receptor antagonists against nausea in humans although there is an anecdotal report that a V_{1a} antagonist was ineffective in motion (see [66]). Although the above studies are all consistent with an intimate role for AVP in the pathogenesis of nausea, it must be noted that there are stimuli which evoked nausea (oral ipecacuanha [122], mild motion [87]) but in which there was no change in [AVP] and a study of patients with idiopathic diabetes insipidus in which nausea was evoked by apomorphine [122]. These studies do not exclude involvement of AVP in the genesis of nausea but do indicate that there are other mechanisms.

The human studies are consistent with studies in animals with an emetic reflex (dog, ferret, monkey) in which a range of stimuli (including apomorphine, abdominal vagal afferent stimulation, cholecystokinin, cisplatin, copper sulphate, lithium chloride) have been shown to produce a dose-related increase plasma AVP (but not oxytocin) either prior to the onset of emesis or in animals showing behavioural changes argued to be an indication of nausea or malaise ([154], for refs.).

If AVP does increase in association with the onset of nausea, what could be its role? A rise in AVP to conserve fluid and stimulate thirst prior to an anticipated loss of fluid by vomiting would be an appropriate adaptive response, and the absence of an equivalent change in rodents that do not vomit is supportive, but the levels of AVP measured in most studies are manyfold greater than those required for a maximal antidiuretic effect by an action at the renal V_2 receptor. The splanchnic vascular bed is sensitive to the vasoconstrictor (V_1) effects of AVP [45], and this would reduce the absorption of a "toxin" from the small intestine [156], and a concomitant decrease in hepatic portal vein flow would buffer the concentration of any absorbed toxin to which the liver was exposed. Intravenous infusion of AVP in humans induces nausea (<5 min), but the reported nausea preceded GMA disturbances (>5 min) in the same subjects [24] suggesting that AVP could be causing nausea via direct activation of vagal afferents or the area postrema. However, in vection studies tachyarrhythmias preceded the onset of reported nausea by about 3 min, and the onset of nausea coincided with a significant rise in AVP (and plasma epinephrine) [178]. The authors of the latter study concluded that it was the gastric dysrhythmias, caused by changes in the autonomic outflow to the stomach, that provided the signal for central secretion of vasopressin. Nausea, plasma AVP and GMA are clearly interrelated, but at present the relatively poor temporal resolution of measurement of each parameter combined with a lack of data on the concentration of AVP required to evoke GMA or motility changes in comparison to the concentration required to evoke nausea makes it hard to unpick what has been referred to as a "noxious trio" [91]. Final resolution of the relationships may have to await studies comparing the efficacy of selective vasopressin receptor antagonists against nausea and the GMA.

Although we have focused on AVP, changes have been reported in a number of other hormones following an emetic stimulus in humans and associated with nausea and these include the following: Pancreatic polypeptide increased following apomorphine in subjects reporting nausea and may be indicative of an increase in vagal efferent drive to the pancreas [50]; plasma epinephrine (adrenalin) increases during vection with levels higher in subjects reporting nausea and the level remained elevated during the recovery period [178]. Although administration of epinephrine can

induce nausea, it appears likely that the increase is more an indication of the perceived stressful nature of vection. Cortisol also increased towards the end of the
period of exposure to vection (at the time AVP was declining) and continued to
increase in recovery [178], and ACTH secretion is reported in subjects given ipecacuanha [124].

Whilst attention has focused on hormones that have their level increased in association with nausea, there are reports of a decrease such as in cortisol in patients
undergoing chemotherapy [115] and ghrelin in volunteers experiencing visually
induced motion sickness [49]. It is argued that hormones whose actions may oppose
the factors mediating nausea are withdrawn as part of the mechanisms generating
nausea, and for both cortisol and ghrelin, it can be argued that their presence (especially at higher concentrations) would be likely to reduce nausea.

2.4.2   *The Autonomic Nervous System and the Stomach*

Associated with nausea, there is an overall increase in sympathetic nervous system
activity and a decrease in vagal drive although the latter does not apply to the
abdominal vagal efferent fibres supplying the enteric inhibitory neurones responsible for proximal gastric relaxation and inhibition of contractile activity [49]. The
changes in autonomic outflow and resulting peripheral responses should be regarded
as components of the activation of the central pathways at a threshold sufficient to
evoke nausea, but preparatory for vomiting, should the stimulus persist or increase
in intensity. The changes in GMA resulting from the reciprocal changes in sympathetic and parasympathetic outflow (possibly enhanced by vasopressin secretion)
appear to lag behind reported nausea by a few minutes, but they do correlate with
nausea intensity although this could simply be because the sensation and the autonomic outflow have a common central origin. Although the GMA changes appear to
follow reports of nausea (vection studies) as the events occurring in stomach wall at
the time nausea is first reported are not known, we should be cautious in dismissing
a causal link, but the questions remain of what the changes could be and how they
would be signalled to the brain. The relationship between gastric motility and nausea is not clear [143] as although nausea induced by vection is associated with relaxation of the proximal stomach and a reduction of antral contractile activity, there
does not appear to be a relationship to symptom severity [47, 144]. However, delayed
gastric emptying is frequently associated with nausea (and vomiting), and symptoms pass when the disorder is treated [143] and gastric antral distension causes
nausea [94]. Although it is unlikely that when nausea is evoked by vection, motion
or the area postrema, the sensation arises initially by detection of gastric motility or
GMA changes, there is no reason why when such changes have occurred as part of
the autonomic changes accompanying nausea, they should not reinforce the sensation via activation of vagal afferents. If an ingested toxin has directly or indirectly
(e.g. via a vago-vagal reflex) produced a delay in gastric emptying, then the nausea
is most likely to arise by activation of vagal afferents projecting to the brainstem.

Monitoring of the autonomic outflows during nausea has shed some light on the "wave-like" nature of nausea by showing that an increased perception of nausea was associated with an increased sympathetic and a decreased parasympathetic activity [88, 93] raising the possibility that the wave-like nature reflects changes in the central autonomic tone during which perception is heightened and lowered [5].

2.4.3   The Brain

Irrespective of the initiating signal, the final step is the activation of a pathway in the brain leading to the genesis of a sensation classified by the individual as nausea. Identification of the pathways within the brain by which the sensation is generated is critical to identification of drugs targeted against nausea and the concomitant autonomic and endocrine changes. fMRI studies in healthy volunteers using vection as the stimulus have identified nausea-related increases in activity in the anterior insula, anterior/mid-cingulate, inferior frontal and middle occipital gyri and medial prefrontal cortex [49, 88, 120], but nausea VAS scores have also been negatively correlated with activity in the cerebellar tonsil, declive, culmen, lingual gyrus, cuneus and left posterior cingulate gyrus [49]. The differential changes in the anterior (increase activity) and posterior cingulate (decrease activity) reported by [49] are particularly interesting as the anterior is involved in control of sympathetic outflow, whereas the posterior is involved in parasympathetic outflow, so the changes are consistent with the altered pattern of autonomic outflow described during nausea (see option 2 above). Using magnetic source imaging, the nausea induced by ingested ipecacuanha was associated with inferior frontal gyrus activity, and the effect was reduced by ondansetron [104, 105]. We are only aware of a single brain imaging study (PET) in cancer patients, and this showed that during delayed emesis severe nausea was associated with an increase in the anterior hypothalamus, anterior cingulate gyrus, thalamus and vermis but a decreased activity in the pons and substantia nigra [56]. Brain imaging studies are clearly in their infancy and in combination with studies to identify the neurotransmitters in the key nuclei offer a tractable approach to identification of drugs targeting specifically nausea irrespective of the cause. Both nausea and vomiting have been induced by discrete electrical stimulation of the human brain in the anterior cingulate cortex and the frontal lobes [38, 148], and the development of more refined non-invasive techniques for brain stimulation will enable the findings from the brain imaging studies to be verified.

2.5   The Physiology of Retching and Vomiting

The purpose of retching and vomiting is to eject the contents, which are presumed to be contaminated, forcibly from the stomach. The mechanical events leading to this expulsion involve specific patterns of motor activity in the striated muscle of the diaphragm, thorax and abdomen and the smooth muscle of the stomach and small intestine driven by the autonomic and somatic divisions of the peripheral nervous system coordinated in the brainstem (see [98] for a rare description of vomiting in humans). Many of the muscles and the central nervous system pathways regulating them that are involved in retching and vomiting are also involved in normal respiration as well as modified respiratory events such as gagging, coughing, sneezing, yawning and straining during defaecation so the coordinated acts of retching and vomiting are an example of "motor programme switching". Retching and vomiting are physically very intense events: there are reports of rib fractures and displaced vertebrae, tears to the oesophagus because of rapid distension by vomitus and wound dehiscence if there has been recent surgery to the abdomen or craniofacial area because of the rapid rise in abdominal and thoracic pressure (estimated to be ~200 mmHg). Additionally, vomiting is demeaning to the patient and worrying to relatives, the odour of vomitus is unpleasant to staff and other patients and vomitus itself can be a source of infection (*Helicobacter pylori*, norovirus). The risk of vomiting prevents the use of medication in tablet form even if nausea permits this although patches and buccal formulations may circumvent this. Protracted vomiting leads to alkalaemia and compromised nutrition.

2.5.1 Pre-expulsion

A number of preparatory changes have occurred in the body prior to the onset of retching and vomiting once the emetic pathways have begun to be stimulated, but the threshold for the induction of vomiting has not been reached and will be summarised here; some of the changes in gut motility have been associated with, but not causally related to, the genesis of the sensation of nausea as described above. The physiological changes largely reflect changes in the autonomic nervous system.

2.5.1.1 Skin

Cold sweating (particularly forehead, forearm, dorsal surface of hand) and a pallid skin (particularly face) are frequently reported to occur in subjects reporting nausea, but there are relatively few detailed studies of this phenomenon, and we are only aware of one study in patients undergoing chemotherapy [114]. These superficial changes are an indication of an increase in sympathetic outflow to the cutaneous vasculature (α-adrenoceptor) and the sweat glands (muscarinic acetylcholine receptors), a combination that is unusual as normally thermally induced sweating would be accompanied by vasodilatation mediated by a decrease in sympathetic constrictor tone. Cutaneous blood flow may also be influenced by plasma vasopressin acting on V_1 receptors, but the effects may be complex as depending upon the concentration, vasopressin may also dilate some vascular beds such as those in the skeletal muscle of the forearm via V_2 receptors [76]; vasodilatation of the forearm has been reported following apomorphine and during motion sickness (Ehrlich and Wallisch 1943, cited [10, 155]).

Specific pattern of cutaneous blood flow changes in animals exposed to a motion stimulus or given emetic drug has been reported [119]. Cutaneous blood flow and sweating are usually related to thermoregulation, and a sensation of feeling hot or a desire for cool air has been reported in association with motion sickness [119] and subjects given apomorphine [23]; these subjective feelings have not been well studied as nausea is the predominating sensation. Further studies of thermoregulation are warranted particularly in patients undergoing chemotherapy as sweating after chemotherapy and feeling warm or hot all over after the last treatment are factors correlated with the probability of anticipatory nausea and vomiting [84].

2.5.1.2 Cardiovascular System

The focus has been on heart rate variability, cardiac vagal tone and respiratory sinus arrhythmia rather than the increase in heart rate or blood pressure changes *per se* because of the information that can be obtained about relative changes in sympathetic and parasympathetic (vagal) efferent outflow with a high temporal resolution. Overall there is a reduction in parasympathetic activity and an increase in sympathetic activity although the majority of data has been obtained during studies of visually induced motion sickness (e.g. [48, 49]). Morrow showed in patients receiving chemotherapy (cisplatin/carboplatin) that there is an increase in heart rate variability reaching a peak ~2 h before nausea was reported but which had decreased from the peak at the time nausea was reported [113]. Morrow also showed that the number of "abnormal" tests of autonomic nervous system function (cardiovascular) was greater in chemotherapy patients who would subsequently have a relatively high level of nausea [116]. Changes in the autonomic tone to the heart have been generalised to the stomach to explain the GMA changes. Caution should be exercised as whilst the activity in the gastric vagal preganglionic efferents supplying the enteric cholinergic neurones is decreased, the drive to the preganglionic vagal efferents supplying the enteric neurones releasing inhibitory transmitters to relax the gastric muscle is increased. For the intestinal retrograde giant contraction (see below) to occur, vagal drive to intestinal cholinergic neurones is increased so when describing autonomic changes generalisations should be avoided.

2.5.1.3 Digestive Tract

The gastric fundus and body are relaxed and antral contractile activity is suppressed (see [154] for refs). The net effect is to delay gastric emptying which confines presumed contaminated material to the stomach where because of the presence of tight intercellular junctions absorption is low in comparison to the intestine and slowing emptying will reduce the peak plasma concentration of any toxin absorbed from the intestine. Additionally, it is proposed that the relaxation of the proximal stomach places it in the most efficient location for compression during the act of vomiting. The reduction of gastric motility is due to a *decrease* in the drive in the preganglionic vagal efferent axons that supply postganglionic cholinergic enteric neurones and an *increase* in the drive to the vagal preganglionic efferents supplying postganglionic enteric neurones releasing inhibitory neurotransmitters (nitric oxide, vasoactive intestinal peptide). The reduction in vagal cholinergic drive contributes to the reduction in gastric acid secretion which arguably blunts the impact of acid vomitus on dentition and the oesophagus and in combination with the increased salivation (parasympathetically mediated) and swallowing often (but not always; see [144]) reported in nauseated subjects or prior to vomiting. An increase in sympathetic activity contributes to the reduction in gastric motility and secretion, but the major effect of the sympathetic system is to reduce gastric and intestinal blood flow with the latter argued to be to further reduce the possibility of toxin absorption.

2.5.2   Expulsion

The last event that occurs prior to the onset of the externally visible acts of retching and vomiting is the occurrence of a retrograde giant contraction (RGC) in the small intestine (see [154] for refs). This forceful contraction (~80 % larger than phase III of the MMC) originates in the mid-small intestine and sweeps towards the stomach and in some cases continues into the antrum. The function of the RGC is presumed to be to propel intestinal contents that may contain toxin into the stomach for ejection. The intestinal contents are alkaline (pancreatic juice) and will help to buffer gastric contents, but as the gall bladder contracts prior to the onset of vomiting, bile is also likely to be present. The RGC requires an intact vagal efferent innervation and can be blocked by atropine showing it is mediated by acetylcholine acting on a muscarinic receptor. Using graded doses of emetics such as apomorphine, it is possible to induce proximal gastric relaxation and a RGC without retching and vomiting ensuing, but if they do, then retching does not begin until the RGC reaches the stomach. It is likely that the point at which a person perceives vomiting as being imminent (a sensation different from nausea?) and may adopt a characteristic posture is when the RGC is initiated possibly reinforced by distension of the stomach by intestinal contents. Even if gastric relaxation and the RGC are blocked, retching and vomiting can still occur so neither represents a target for a drug to block vomiting. Retching involves contraction of the crural and costal regions of the diaphragm under the influence of the phrenic nerve and the rectus abdominis and external intercostals under the influence of spinal motor neurones. Little is known of the factors regulating the number of retches preceding a vomit although animal studies (ferret) suggest that this is inversely related to gastric volume [4]. The primary change to permit vomiting is that the crural region of the diaphragm that contributes to the anti-reflux barrier between the stomach and oesophagus is inhibited, but the remainder of the diaphragm and abdominal muscles contract more intensely in longer duration bursts each coincident with forceful oral expulsion of gastric contents with a propulsive force of ~200 mmHg. The pudendal nerves tighten the urethral and anal sphincters during vomiting. The stomach itself plays a primarily passive role in vomiting as it is compressed by the diaphragm and abdominal muscles. Blocking retching and vomiting by a drug acting at the peripheral motor terminals in the diaphragm and abdominal muscles is possible using curare-like drugs, but of course breathing would also be prevented and this illustrates why anti-emetic drugs are either targeted at the central integrative mechanisms (e.g. NK_1 receptor antagonists) or the initiating input pathways (e.g. $5\text{-}HT_3$ receptor antagonists) (see below for details).

2.5.3 Between Emetic Episodes

Almost nothing is known about what happens in the gut between episodes of emesis, what determines the interval between episodes (hence the intensity of emesis) and what determines the overall duration of the emetic response. For substances such as morphine, the duration is determined by the overall plasma level and concentration, but for others such as cisplatin, the emesis continues long after plasma levels have subsided. A crucial question is at what point normal patterns of gastrointestinal motility resume as this is critical for the patient's ability to eat. There is also a more general issue of when the range of autonomic nervous system changes which occur in association with nausea and during the pre-expulsion and expulsion phases reverts to normal after the end of the last emetic episode.

2.6 Inputs: How Are Nausea and Vomiting Induced?

The gastrointestinal tract, the area postrema (in the fourth ventricle) and the vestibular labyrinths are the major structures which when activated by adequate stimuli cause induction of nausea and/or vomiting. In many ways these sites reflect the hierarchically organised system by which the body defends itself against ingested toxins. Understanding the way in which chemotherapeutic agents, other medications given as part of cancer treatment and cancer itself interact with these structures is critical to both understanding the origin of CINV and providing insights into current and future anti-emetic therapies. In addition, to these inputs consideration also needs to be given to the pathways implicated in the genesis of anticipatory nausea and vomiting. As a background to the sections below describing in detail the mechanism of acute, delayed and anticipatory chemotherapy-induced nausea and vomiting and the sites of anti-emetics, we will first review what is known about these key inputs and central integration from general studies of emesis.

2.6.1   The Tongue and Pharynx

These structures are not considered as "classical" sites from which the central emetic pathways can be activated but the gustatory system and particularly the identification of bitter-tasting substances form part of the toxin-detecting system (see above). Taste buds detecting bitter substances supplied by glossopharyngeal and vagal (see also below) afferents project to the nucleus tractus solitarius in the brainstem. Controlled studies have demonstrated that nausea accompanied by characteristic changes in gastric myoelectric activity can be induced by application of bitter-tasting chemicals to the tongue [129]. More general links between bitter taste sensitivity and nausea come from studies showing an increased propensity to motion sickness in individuals with high sensitivity to bitter stimuli [175] and a positive relationship between hyperemesis gravidarum and bitter taste perception [152]. In view of these findings, the early reports of rapid-onset (~30 min) bitter taste associated with some chemotherapeutic agents (cyclophosphamide, methotrexate, 5-FU chemotherapy) and which some patients considered the cause of their emesis [51] may need to be re-evaluated as clearly chemotherapeutic agents have the capability of activating bitter taste buds and this could also be responsible for increased salivation, swallowing and lip licking which have variably been reported to accompany nausea [7]. The proteins involved in the detection of bitter-tasting substances are members of the type 2 taste receptor (T2R) family with molecular and functional studies showing expression and physiological effects in the gastrointestinal tract (including 5-hydroxytryptamine containing enterochromaffin cells) and airway [52]. The molecular interactions of cytotoxic drugs with enterochromaffin cells are reviewed in detail below, but studies of the binding of cytotoxic drugs to the ~25 members of the T2R family would be of interest and may give insights into predicting emetic liability.

2.6.2   The Gastrointestinal Tract and Visceral Afferents

Once contaminated food has been swallowed, prompt detection whilst the toxin is still in the gut lumen provides the last opportunity for ejection in bulk by vomiting or diarrhoea before the toxins can damage the epithelium by prolonged contact and are absorbed. Emesis can be induced rapidly once a threshold is reached as illustrated by the observation that emesis can be triggered in <1 min by continuous electrical stimulation of the abdominal vagal afferents in the ferret [4]. Once toxins are in the blood stream, they may be metabolised by the liver and excreted via the kidneys, but when in the circulation, the potential for damage, especially of the brain, is considerably increased and vomiting will have no effect on plasma concentrations of already absorbed toxin. Information from the gut is signalled to the central nervous system via afferent axons travelling in either sympathetic (splanchnic) or parasympathetic (predominantly vagus but also sacral nerves not considered here) nerve trunks which also contain efferent axons influencing a range of gut functions (motility, blood flow, exocrine and endocrine secretions).

2.6.2.1   Abdominal Vagal Afferents

There are two main populations of vagal afferents (see [22] for additional details), and both have their cell body of origin in the nodose ganglion and terminate in the nucleus tractus solitarius with some limited animal data for additional projections to the area postrema:

Mechanoreceptors

These are afferent axons with terminations (intraganglionic laminar endings; IGLE) in the myenteric ganglia and signal both contraction and distension of the gut muscle with the density higher in the oesophagus, stomach and small intestine than in the first part of the colon [22]. These afferents are implicated in induction of nausea and vomiting in at least two ways; firstly distension of gut regions such as the gastric antrum and the duodenum which are not regions of the gut specialised for accommodation are sites from which nausea and vomiting can be induced; secondly, if accommodation (relaxation) mechanisms are impaired in the proximal stomach due to selective loss of inhibitory (nitric oxide, vasoactive intestinal peptide) enteric neurones (e.g. diabetic neuropathy; chronic effect of cisplatin), then wall tension even in response to a normal-size meal may activate the afferents sufficiently to induce nausea [143]. The stomach normally maintains a low level of motility so the mechanoreceptors always signal a low level of activity; hence it is possible that motor quiescence such as occurs in the stomach in association with nausea may itself constitute a signal. The IGLE terminals of the afferents have a number of receptors that can modulate their sensitivity (e.g. inhibitory $GABA_B$ and ghrelin; excitatory glutamate), and these receptors are a potential target for drugs to treat gastroesophageal reflux, obesity as well as nausea and vomiting depending on the cause [143].

Mucosal Afferents

This population of afferents found in the oesophagus, stomach and small intestine monitors various features of the luminal environment [22] including pH, osmolarity and chemical stimuli including nutrients (see below) and also responds to abrasion of the mucosa such as might occur in the stomach during digestion of pieces of meat and compression of the mucosa as may occur in lumen occluding contractions as can occur during phase III of the migrating motor complex or intestinal retrograde giant contraction. The anatomical correlate of the mucosal afferent is a vagal afferent axon terminating in close proximity to one member of the family of enteroendocrine cells in the mucosa. In response to a luminal stimulus, the enteroendocrine cell releases via exocytosis one or more mediators which can modulate (stimulate or inhibit) vagal afferent activity via receptors located on the vagal afferent terminal, and in some cases (peptides) the substances can enter the hepatic portal vein and, provided they survive plasma, hepatic and pulmonary metabolism, enter the systemic circulation and act as hormones elsewhere in the body including the area postrema in the brainstem (see below). Physiologically the enteroendocrine cells respond to stimuli in the gut lumen, but if a systemic agent triggers the exocytotic process to release a mediator, then this substance will in effect have the same effect as the luminal stimulus, but the effect is likely to be magnified as the systemic stimulus will act simultaneously on all cells in the gut sensitive to it, whereas a natural luminal stimulus would be expected to have a more localised action. There are several populations of enteroendocrine cells containing a diverse range of mediators but the enterochromaffin cells (see below), the location of ~90 % of the 5-HT in the body is perhaps the best known releasing its 5-HT to activate 5-HT$_3$ receptors on the vagal afferents terminating in close proximity [16]. It must be emphasised that this released 5-HT acts locally in a high concentration and that 5-HT entering the hepatic portal vein is either metabolised or taken up by platelets so the 5-HT from the EC cells does not act as a circulating hormone. Other substances found in enteroendocrine cells include cholecystokinin (CCK), glucagon-like peptide-1 (GLP-1) and peptide YY (PYY) which have been implicated in induction of satiety by a local effect on the vagal afferents but can also have an endocrine role with an effect on the circumventricular organs (including the area postrema). Studies in humans and animals have shown that CCK, GLP-1 and PYY or synthetic analogues have the potential to induce nausea and vomiting (see [5], for refs). The enteroendocrine cells and the associated vagal afferents have an important role in the regulation of food intake and the sensation of satiety, the control of gut motility and secretion in addition to being part of the body's defensive system by induction of nausea and vomiting by luminal chemicals (e.g. copper sulphate, hypertonic saline) and viruses (e.g. rotavirus, [68]).

2.6.2.2 Splanchnic Afferents

These afferents have their peripheral terminals in proximity to or on blood vessels (arteries and second-order arterioles) in the gut wall, with cell bodies in the dorsal root ganglia (DRG) and central terminations in the dorsal horn of the spinal cord. Although responding to stretch and contraction, the sensitivity is less than that of the mechanoreceptive vagal afferents, they also respond to noxious stimuli, reduced mesenteric blood flow, ischaemia and hypoxia [22]. There is little evidence that they are able to directly induce retching and vomiting in contrast to abdominal vagal afferents, but as pain is one consequence of their activation, they could be involved in the sensation of nausea that accompanies intense pain (e.g. biliary colic) with the second-order projections in the spinothalamic pathway project collaterals to the nucleus tractus solitarius and the parabrachial nucleus providing the substrate. In patients with post-operative nausea and vomiting and pain following abdominal surgery, treating the pain reduced the nausea [3]. As these afferents respond to reduced blood flow and ischaemia, they could be involved in genesis of the sensation of nausea associated with mesenteric ischaemia, but it should also be recalled that gut blood flow is reduced (as indicated by mucosal pallor) in association with nausea and could contribute to genesis of the sensation. Although the splanchnic afferents are probably not involved in reflex induction of emesis, they may have a role in nausea but this requires direct investigation.

2.6.3   The Area Postrema

The human brain has eight circumventricular organs (CVO), all of which have the common feature of being regions where the blood-brain barrier is relatively permeable because of the presence of fenestrated endothelia [19, 95, 96, 100, 177]. The area postrema is the only CVO located in the fourth ventricle and is the only one (to date) implicated in induction of nausea and vomiting. The area postrema was implicated in induction of emesis from animal studies (initially dog and cat; [19] for review) showing that ablation blocked the emetic response to some (but not all) emetic drugs given systemically or applied topically. This ability to detect specific substances in the circulation and to evoke emesis led to it being called "the chemoreceptor trigger zone", and whilst this is useful shorthand, the use of this terminology encouraged the erroneous view, particularly with chemotherapeutic drugs, that agents present in the circulation must be inducing emesis via this site. The area postrema should be regarded as "a" chemoreceptor trigger zone rather than "the" chemoreceptor trigger zone. The area postrema has been surgically ablated in humans [97] in an attempt to treat intractable vomiting, but the efficacy of the procedure was tested using administration of the dopamine D_2 receptor agonist apomorphine as it is commonly used to test the same lesion in animal studies; this is a rare example of where the same lesion has been compared with the same emetic challenge in humans and animals. In humans chronic nausea was associated with neurenteric cyst of the area postrema [106], and intractable vomiting is a symptom of aquaporin-4 autoimmunity acting on the area postrema (neuromyelitis optica; [132, 135]) supporting its involvement in pathways.

Related to emesis the area postrema has also been implicated in genesis of learned food aversions. Although the focus here is on the effects of exogenous agents, the CVOs are variably sensitive to a range of endogenous hormones implicated in the regulation of food intake (CCK, GLP-1, TNF-α), blood pressure control and salt and water intake (AII, AVP; [19, 96]; Price, 2008). The CVOs therefore contribute to homeostasis and are able to influence behaviour. Although the area postrema is implicated in a number of functions, we know little of how the concentration of a substance acting on the AP cells is translated into a graded response of nausea followed by vomiting at a higher concentration. A diverse range of substances can affect the area postrema, but we do not know the full spectrum of receptors present on AP cells or indeed which cells in the AP are involved in responding to which substances. Whilst responses to exogenous application of chemicals known to be endogenous transmitters or hormones can be reconciled in terms of the presence of a diverse receptor (e.g. AII [AT_{1A}], CCK $_1$, GLP-1, ghrelin [GHSR], IL-1, $P2_{X2}$, nAch, TNF-α, AVP [V_1], D_2, enkephalin, PYY [Y1/Y2/Y4]) or ion channel (H^+, K^+, Ca^{++}, [150]) population, it is unclear if, and how, other chemicals (e.g. cisplatin, copper sulphate, imiquimod) where area postrema ablation has been shown to affect their emetic response interact with the area postrema.

2.6.4 The Vestibular System and Vestibulo-Visual Conflicts

Although there is no direct evidence that the vestibular system is implicated in acute or delayed chemotherapy-induced emesis, the sensitivity to motion sickness is correlated with sensitivity to both acute and delayed chemotherapy-induced emesis (e.g. [112, 149]), post-operative nausea and vomiting and pregnancy sickness [21, 174]. The mechanisms underlying the correlations are not fully known, but known projections of the vestibular system to the vestibular nucleus which in turn projects to the nucleus tractus solitarius which is intimately involved in the coordination of the emetic outputs provide a mechanism by which vestibular inputs modulate overall emetic sensitivity. This observation is also consistent with the experience that moving the head exacerbates nausea from non-vestibular causes and reports that acute PONV can be triggered as patients are moved on a trolley from the operating theatre. Drugs with primary efficacy against central muscarinic and H_1 receptors and used for the treatment of motion sickness have some efficacy against emesis induced by chemotherapy, radiotherapy and post-operative nausea and vomiting where there is no evidence for a direct vestibular involvement, but the efficacy could be explained by a reduction in the tonic drive to the nucleus tractus solitarius changing the threshold for other inputs to trigger the system. Although terrestrial motion sickness can be driven purely from the vestibular system, the usual mechanism involves a conflict between the vestibular and visual systems. However, a form of motion sickness (visually induced motion sickness) can be induced in a stationary subject exposed to a scene giving the sensation of self-motion (vection); this induces a conflict between the information received by the brain from the eyes (movement) and the vestibular system (no movement). Whilst there is debate about similarities and differences between "real" and "virtually" induced motion sickness, the latter has a provided a convenient controllable stimulus to study nausea in a laboratory setting, and much of the information about nausea reviewed below comes from such studies (e.g. [49]).

2.6.5 Cortical Inputs

It is clear that unpleasant smells or horrific sights can trigger nausea and vomiting, but the pathways by which this occurs are not known and nor is it known to what extent this may be a culturally determined learned response or a reaction to severe stress. However, it is known that in the context of chemotherapy anticipatory nausea and vomiting can be triggered in susceptible individuals by visual (sight of the oncologist) and olfactory (smell of the disinfectant) cues linked to the environment in which the nausea and vomiting was experienced during the chemotherapy with the response heightened by the stress caused by the anticipation of the next cycle. This classical conditioned response can be reduced by optimal anti-emetic treatment on the first and each cycle of chemotherapy and psychological interventions such as overshadowing.

2.7 Central Integration

The signals from the abdominal vagal afferents, the area postrema and the vestibular system indicating whether nausea and vomiting should result converge in the brainstem in the nucleus tractus solitarius (NTS) and from this major integrative nucleus outputs (not necessarily direct) pass to two main locations (see [58, 154] for refs): (1) brainstem nuclei including the retrofacial nucleus and central respiratory group regulating the spinal output to the phrenic nerve and diaphragm (retching and vomiting), pre-sympathetic neurones in the rostral ventrolateral medulla (heart, arterioles, sweat glands, adrenal gland), salivatory nuclei, dorsal motor vagal nucleus (vagal supply to gut) and nucleus ambiguus (pharynx, larynx, upper oesophagus, heart) and (2) rostral brain including the hypothalamus (AVP secretion), cingulate ("visceromotor" cortex; particularly involved implicated in regulation of ANS outflow) and insular ("interoceptive" cortex) cortex. These and adjacent nuclei (e.g. amygdala) provide a substrate for the behavioural and autonomic changes which accompany nausea as well as the sensory experience.

The critical integrative role of the NTS goes some way to explaining the "broad-spectrum" effects of NK_1 receptor antagonists which have a major site of action here (see [8, 58] for detailed reviews). It is interesting to consider at which point on the "output" side of the NTS the signals for nausea to more rostral structures and for vomiting to other brainstem nuclei diverge as drugs targeted at this divergent point should be equally efficacious against nausea and vomiting initiated by inputs to the NTS.

2.8 Endogenous Anti-emetic Mechanisms

There are several pieces of evidence for endogenous mechanisms capable of reducing the vomiting and possibly nausea (c.f. endogenous anti-nociceptive pathways). Understanding how these endogenous pathways are activated to suppress and deactivated to facilitate emesis is of obvious relevance to identifying novel approaches to anti-emesis.

2.8.1   Pulmonary Vagal Afferents

Electrical stimulation of the abdominal vagal afferents readily induced emesis, but stimulation of the cervical vagus containing the afferents from the gut *en route* to the brainstem and afferents from thoracic structures does not. It is hypothesised that vagal pulmonary afferents are responsible for this effect by "neuroinhibitory stabilisation" of the brainstem emesis network [180]. In addition to emesis induced by abdominal vagal afferent stimulation and emesis induced by xylazine acting via the area postrema, motion-induced emesis can also be blocked by cervical vagal afferent simulation. In humans deep breathing is known to alleviate the sensation of nausea, and the activation of pulmonary afferents modulating brainstem pathways provides a plausible explanation although this has not been investigated directly. The availability of transcutaneous and implantable vagal nerve stimulators should allow direct investigation of vagal nerve stimulation as a therapeutic option particularly if the pulmonary afferents can be stimulated selectively without affecting normal respiratory control.

2.8.2   Brain Mechanisms

Rimonabant is an antagonist at cannabinoid receptors and can induce nausea suggesting that they are blocking tonically active endogenous pathways that are suppressing nausea [130]. In addition naloxone can reduce the threshold dose required for apomorphine or motion to induce emesis [2, 90]. Further support for endogenous inhibitory pathways comes from the observation that a number of anti-emetic agents, often with some degree of "broad-spectrum" activity, are agonists with actions at mu opioid, cannabinoid$_1$, 5-hydroxytryptamine$_{1A}$ and TRPV$_1$ receptors [5].

2.9   Acute and Delayed CINV: Mechanism, Pathways and Aspects of Anti-emetic Pharmacology

The above pathways provide a framework within which to discuss the mechanisms by which cytotoxic drugs act to induce nausea and vomiting. Of necessity, we will need to rely on data from animal models for mechanisms as it is not feasible to undertake comparable lesion studies in patients (area postrema ablation; truncal vagotomy) although studies in which similar pharmacological agents have been studied in animals and patients provide support for similar mechanisms. Extrapolating from drug effects in animals to humans often provides the only insight into mechanisms and pathways in humans, and in many cases we may have to accept that we will never know the detailed mechanisms in humans in the same way as animals. The majority of studies have investigated cisplatin or cisplatin-containing regimes so these will be the focus of the discussion, but differences and discrepancies with other cytotoxics will be highlighted. The complexity of the effects of cytotoxic drugs on the body should not be overlooked and is well illustrated by a microarray study of the stomach in the rat showing that within 48 h of a single injection of cisplatin there was a greater than twofold change in >1,000 genes and greater than tenfold change in >20 genes [64].

2.9.1 Before Chemotherapy

The emetic response to a particular chemotherapy agent will be determined by patient-dependent predisposing factors as well as the chemotherapy agent itself. Although the mechanism underlying some of the factors predisposing to an emetic response such as younger age, female sex and abstention from alcohol is unclear, others such as a emetic history (motion sickness, pregnancy sickness), low pre-chemotherapy nocturnal cortisol [83], an elevated pre-chemotherapy ratio of substance P to 5-hydroxyindoleacetic acid/creatinine in the urine [75] and polymorphisms that may affect the efficacy of 5-HT$_3$ receptor antagonists [9, 20, 158, 165, 166, 181] can readily be explained within our understanding of the neuropharmacology of CINV. Identification of other biomarkers indicative of patient sensitivity to an emetic challenge (e.g. central anti-emetic tone; see section above) will assist in individualising anti-emetic therapy to enhance efficacy. Concomitant medication such as morphine [151] for which the emetic response is also impacted by polymorphisms [157] and prior surgery is also likely to impact on sensitivity. Animal models investigating mechanisms of emesis induced by chemotherapeutic agents have not investigated the impact of a tumour likely to result in the release of pro-emetic/inflammatory mediators. The psychological state of the patient will also impact as anxiety increases the probability of emesis in several situations. In view of these factors (and probably many of which we are not yet aware), it is perhaps unsurprising that patients given the same chemotherapy agents and same anti-emetic may experience quite different outcomes.

2.9.2 Acute Phase of Emesis Induced by Chemotherapy

There have been several attempts to identify a unifying mechanism to explain the emetic effect of cytotoxic drugs with diverse chemical structures and anticancer targets. Harris hypothesised that chemotherapeutic drugs acted to inhibit the synthesis of enzymes responsible for the *metabolism* of enkephalins resulting in an activation of opioid receptors (delta-opioid receptors) and induction of emesis via release of dopamine in the area postrema [69]. Within the same hypothesis, it was thought there was a concurrent inhibition of the *synthesis* of enkephalins with inhibitory actions (via the activation of μ-opioid receptors) at the "vomiting centre" [70]. However, whilst the opioid receptor antagonist, naloxone, is capable of potentiating emesis induced by a number of challenges, the overall hypothesis that chemotherapeutic drugs differentially affect the synthesis/metabolism of endogenous opioids is difficult to rationalise [55, 140] and has been superseded by a focus of how chemotherapy may affect the function synthesis, metabolism and release of 5-HT and substance P driven mainly by studies investigating the mechanism of 5-HT$_3$ and NK$_1$ receptor antagonists. In the limited space it is not possible to review all the original evidence supporting the current model of the mechanisms underlying CINV, but the following reviews cover the key issues and also differences of opinion [6, 8, 32, 34, 73, 107].

Although the "enkephalin hypothesis" is no longer current, it did raise the concept of a "unifying initiating mechanism" and cautioned against confusing the primary effect of the cytotoxic drugs at the point initiating emesis with secondary neurotransmitter pathways activated as a consequence (see [70]). Identifying primary and secondary effects remains an issue and is at the core of understanding how cytotoxic drugs induce emesis and how anti-emetics can interfere with the consequential pathway activation.

Using cisplatin as an example, we will summarise the evidence from both animals and humans for the "5-HT–SP hypothesis", but we emphasise that this is still a working hypothesis and, although consistent with the majority of evidence, there are gaps and unresolved issues which it must be recognised may never be filled or reconciled particularly by studies in humans. Bearing in mind that the cytotoxic drug is being administered to a patient whose emetic pathways may be "primed" by the presence of a cancer, prior surgery, emetic history, genetically determined endogenous factors and concomitant medication, what is the sequence of events that lead to the activation of the input pathways described above leading to induction of acute nausea and vomiting?

2.9.2.1 The Latent Period and the Enterochromaffin Cell–Vagal Afferent Unit

For all emetic stimuli, there is a delay (latent period) between initiation of the stimulus and the onset of a response (nausea and/or vomiting). For some cytotoxic drugs such as cyclophosphamide, a component of the latency is contributed by the time for hepatic metabolism to phosphoramide mustard and acrolein; the former is known to be emetic but the emetic properties of the latter are not known. Cisplatin enters cells in its di-chloro form, but once in the cells where there is a lower concentration of chloride ions compared to the plasma, the two chloride ions are substituted for water by hydrolysis with the t$_{1/2}$ for this reaction being ~6 h [161]. The emetogenic potential (proportion of patients experiencing emesis in the absence of effective anti-emetic prophylaxis) of a number of cytotoxic drugs (carmustine, cisplatin, cyclophosphamide, doxorubicin and methotrexate) is dependent upon the dose and rate of administration as illustrated by cisplatin where the acute response can be reduced by using a slow infusion [86]. Studies in the ferret and dog have shown that the latency of acute emesis to cisplatin is inversely related to dose [4] and in man high doses can have a latency of a few hours comparable to the 1–2 h observed in dog and ferret (ibid). So what is happening in this time period before emesis begins? The enteroendocrine cells in the gut and particularly the 5-HT-containing enterochromaffin (EC) cells are the primary target for the cytotoxic drugs during the acute phase of CINV. It is often assumed that cisplatin enters the EC cells by passive diffusion, but there is growing evidence from other tissues for a contribution by transport proteins with the tissue distribution of such transported implicated in renal toxicity and ototoxicity [27, 101]. The presence or otherwise of cytotoxic drug transporters (including efflux) on EC cells would be of interest and could explain why such cells have such a high sensitivity to cytotoxic drugs.

What is happening when cytotoxic drugs enter the EC cell? Based largely on animal studies, it is proposed that cisplatin and other cytotoxic drugs cause the production of free radicals in the EC cells and these induce the influx of Ca^{++} into the cells via L-type Ca^{++}channels triggering exocytotic release of 5-HT. This hypothesis is supported by studies showing induction of emesis by free radical generators and blockade of cisplatin-induced acute emesis by antioxidants [18, 67, 162, 163]. It would be interesting to compare the ability of cytotoxic drugs to generate free radicals in EC cells with their emetogenicity. The release of 5-HT by exocytosis from EC cells has also been implicated in emesis induced by rotavirus and staphylococcal enterotoxin [68, 81], observations consistent with the proposed defensive role of the gut epithelium. Although we focus on exocytosis triggered by free radicals, 5-HT release from EC cells is also under neural control, and hence an acute effect of a cytotoxic drug on enteric neurones could also be involved (see [107] for review) although this does not appear to be the main mechanism. The release of 5-HT from the EC cells is subject to a number of modulatory endocrine and neural (e.g. enteric nervous system) influences which may themselves be influenced by cisplatin and other cytotoxic drugs [111, 133]. For example, in the least shrew intestinal endocannabinoid levels are reduced within 30–60 min of cisplatin administration [33].

Evidence for the release of 5-HT by cytotoxic drugs comes from animal studies showing effects on isolated EC or EC-like tumour cells or intestine in vitro [109, 145], measurement of ileal dialysate in dogs given cisplatin [59] and measurement of blood and urinary 5-hydroxyindole acetic acid (5-HIAA, a metabolite of 5-HT produced by the action of monoamine oxidase (MAO) as the 5-HT passes into the liver via the hepatic portal vein) in patients undergoing chemotherapy [25, 30, 31, 41, 74, 176]. The studies by Cubeddu [30, 31] also measured plasma chromogranin A (CGA) the vesicle storage protein which is co-released with 5-HT and provides an additional marker of EC cell exocytosis [16]. There is no consistent evidence that the plasma concentration of 5-HT rises following chemotherapy, and studies in which increases have been observed may reflect technical differences from measuring a blood sample [12] vs. using intravenous microdialysis [25] particularly as the platelets which are responsible for the uptake of the majority of EC cell released 5-HT are a rich source of 5-HT.

Additional support for the EC cell being the target for cytotoxic drugs comes from showing that depletion of EC cell 5-HT using parachlorophenylalanine markedly reduced the nausea and vomiting in patients treated with cisplatin [1], findings partially supported by studies in the ferret [139].

The 5-HT from the EC cells acts locally on $5-HT_3$ receptors (a ligand-gated ion channel) located on vagal afferents terminating in close proximity, a mechanism readily demonstrated by direct recording from intestinal vagal afferents showing blockade of cisplatin-induced activity by $5-HT_3$ receptor antagonists [44, 80, 107]. In contrast to other 5-HT receptors, the $5-HT_3$ receptor requires a relatively high concentration for activation, >1 μM for $5-HT_3$ vs. 1–10 nM for G-protein-coupled 5-HT receptors [16, 134]. This further emphasises the importance of the release of a "high" concentration of 5-HT acting on receptors located nearby, and it is estimated that the concentration will be >10 nM at 5 μm from the cell.

Additional support for involvement of the vagus comes from the demonstration that surgical section of the abdominal vagi (either with or without concomitant greater splanchnic nerve section) abolishes or reduces the emetic response to cisplatin in several species (ferret, [71]; house musk shrew, [118]; dog, [61]; monkey, [60]). The involvement of the abdominal vagal afferents in acute CINV is consistent with the role of the EC cell – vagus in detection of ingested toxins, and it is also relevant that the abdominal vagus is implicated in the acute emetic response to total body radiation [4] which is also sensitive to $5-HT_3$ receptor antagonists.

Although we have focused on the role of 5-HT from the EC cells in driving the response via the activation of $5-HT_3$ receptors located on the vagal afferent terminals, other substances released either from the EC, enteroendocrine or mast cells can act on receptors located on the vagal afferent terminals to both drive and sensitise/desensitise the response to 5-HT, and vice versa. Of particular interest is substance P, and an interaction was hypothesised to explain why an NK_1 receptor antagonist reduced vagal afferent activation by 5-HT and a $5-HT_3$ receptor antagonist reduced the response to substance P [108]. These studies are of interest in light of the recent studies on the molecular effects of palonosetron and "crosstalk" between NK_1 and $5-HT_3$ receptors [136]. An action on the peripheral vagal NK_1 receptors could contribute to the anti-emetic effect of NK_1 receptor antagonists in CINV, but the weight of evidence favours a predominantly central, primarily nucleus tractus solitarius, site of action (see [8] for review) in contrast to the predominantly peripheral site of action for $5-HT_3$ receptor antagonists.

The abdominal vagal afferents have a major role in the regulation of food intake by providing the initial satiety signal and in the regulation of vago-vagal reflexes, motility and secretion. We do not know how the signals for the initiation of the physiological regulatory processes are encoded and processed centrally in comparison to the vagal afferent signals signalling nausea and vomiting.

The above discussion has focused on the activation of abdominal vagal afferents primarily by 5-HT with a likely involvement of other locally released substances (e.g. SP). However, we should not overlook the possibility that the area postrema may also be involved with its role being permissive or facilitating the vagal afferent input. For example, in the dog plasma levels of the peptide YY

(PYY) known to induce emesis increased following cisplatin with a profile that followed emesis [128]; PYY is one of a number of gut peptides that have an emetic potential (e.g. CCK, GLP-1) and are known to act on the area postrema, but there have been insufficient studies of gut hormone profiles following chemotherapy (e.g. see [82]) to provide evidence to include or dismiss this option. It is of course possible that cisplatin could be acting directly on the AP as it rapidly accesses the brainstem although the levels are <20-fold lower than in the plasma at the same time points (house musk shrew, [43]). Whilst neuronal cell bodies in the AP could respond directly to cisplatin and there is evidence from dorsal root ganglia for an increase in excitability caused by cisplatin concentrations in the clinical range and a protective effect of dexamethasone [147], a more likely target is the astrocyte-like cells (glia) with processes surrounding neurones and end-feet contacting the perivascular spaces (i.e. the circulation) which are a prominent feature of the AP [96]. Astrocytes are known to possess the organic cation transporter responsible for uptake of cisplatin, and studies in rat hippocampus have shown binding of cisplatin to rough endoplasmic reticulum in astrocytes with end-feet contacting vessels [182]. The functional consequences of such uptake if it occurred in the AP astrocytes are unknown but could prove a credible mechanism by which cisplatin could modulate the outflow of the AP to the NTS.

If the AP is involved in the acute phase, its role is likely to be facilitatory as overall pathways from the AP to the NTS are not sensitive to 5-HT$_3$ receptor antagonists. However, it is conceivable that in some individuals the AP pathways have a more significant role, and if so, this could explain why 5-HT$_3$ receptor antagonists may be less efficacious in some patients. In these cases NK$_1$ receptor antagonists would be expected to be effective because of the predominant site of action in the NTS [8].

2.9.2.2 Sustaining and Stopping the Acute Emetic Response

The above section describes how the primarily vagal pathways are activated, but it should be appreciated that as the acute phase continues for ~18 h the pathways are being subject to sustained activation. As the entire acute phase is 5-HT$_3$ receptor antagonist sensitive and administration of a 5-HT$_3$ receptor antagonist after vomiting has begun can stop the response within a few minutes in ferrets and humans [15], it is likely that the pathway is being continuously driven and/or sensitised by 5-HT release. The cessation of the acute phase at 18–24 h is not due to depletion of 5-HT [28] so the decline is due to removal of the driving stimulus with a reciprocal change in the capacity of the EC cells to generate and scavenge free radicals being likely mechanisms although the possibility that compensatory mechanisms damping the release of 5-HT is induced. A comparison of cisplatin and cyclophosphamide over 48 h may give insights. As the mechanisms driving the acute phase decline, those responsible for the delayed phase become active but against the background of a central nervous system that has received a continuous emetic drive for ~18 h.

2.9.3   Delayed Phase Induced by Chemotherapy

If the defining feature of the acute phase of cisplatin-induced emesis is the intensity of emesis, the duration of 2–4 days is the hallmark of the delayed phase which begins after a period of little or no emesis around 18–24 h following high-dose cisplatin administration [92]. Although other chemotherapeutic agents such as doxorubicin and cyclophosphamide can induce emesis beyond 24 h in the case of cyclophosphamide, it is rare that this continues beyond 48 h. Whilst the initial differentiation of acute and delayed phases was temporal, there is a growing body of evidence based primarily on the relative efficacy of anti-emetics indicating that they should be regarded as having distinctive mechanisms [73, 138]. Anxiety (probably based upon the experience during the first 24 h) plays some role as urinary noradrenaline levels are predictive of delayed nausea but not emesis [57], and there may also be pharmacokinetic reasons as delayed emesis was more likely to occur in patients with slower cisplatin clearance [131]. However a number of observations provide evidence for different mechanisms. Preclinical studies in several species (see above) demonstrate a major role for the abdominal vagal innervation in the acute phase of cisplatin, and there is evidence that the area postrema is involved in the delayed phase [127], but as we are unlikely to ever have comparable data from humans, mechanisms need to be based on comparing the pharmacological effects of anti-emetics in animals and humans. We propose the following as model that explains a number of observations but which remains to be tested in humans.

The delayed phase is most likely to be due to endogenous processes initiated in the acute phase by administration of the cytotoxic drug as blood levels of the original drug are minimal at 24–48 h. However, it is possible that native cytotoxic drug (e.g. cisplatin) or its metabolite (e.g. phosphoramide mustard for cyclophosphamide) could become sequestered in the area postrema which has a relatively high blood flow and which has been argued to have a countercurrent mechanism capable of concentrating substances in the plasma. Drugs could also reach the nucleus tractus solitarius via fenestrated capillaries known to be present in rodents, but the observation that the delayed phase (ferret, [127]) can be blocked by area postrema ablation suggests that a direct action at the NTS is not the main mechanism involved in delayed emesis.

Animal studies have shown that administration of a single dose of a cisplatin produces a diverse range of changes in the brain and gut including: gene expression (e.g. preprotachykinin-1 [39]), gastrin and somatostatin [173], ghrelin receptor [99], levels of transmitters (e.g. endocannabinoids [33]), 5-HT and dopamine [11, 139], SP [43], gastric neuronal nitric oxide synthase [85], brain oncogenes (e.g. c-fos, [77]), intestinal epithelial absorption [14] and gastrointestinal motility [169, 179]. Although some of these changes may be affected by an anti-emetics (e.g. c-Fos expression in the brain secondary to abdominal vagal afferent activation), many will not. Many of these changes will persist giving multiple potential mechanisms that could contribute to the delayed phase. Whilst AP ablation implicates a systemically released agent, the identity of which is not known, it is highly likely in humans that the delayed phase is contributed to by inflammatory processes (gut and AP) and disturbed gastric motility which provide rational targets for the efficacy of dexamethasone and metoclopramide [138]. It is perhaps unsurprising that NK_1 receptor antagonists are effective in the delayed phase as the primary site of action is in the NTS at the convergence point of the inputs likely to be activated by the above array of changes triggered by cisplatin [8].

It is unlikely that we will know which of the changes described above occurring in animals also occur in patients, and even for the animals we do not know the time taken for recovery, but this could help identify the main factors responsible for the delayed phase. However, it is likely that some of these changes will persist and be in place when patients receive the next course of chemotherapy.

2.9.3.1 Subsequent Cycles

Although we have a reasonable understanding of the mechanisms responsible for acute and delayed chemotherapy-induced emesis on the first cycle, little is known about how (or if) the mechanism differs on subsequent cycles although a reduction in efficacy of anti-emetics with number of cycles is a strong indication of underlying changes. However, Cubeddu (1993) reported in patients that during the acute phase of cisplatin-induced emesis urinary excretion of 5-HIAA during subsequent cycles (combined data from cycles 2, 3 or 4) was the same or higher than those during the first cycle [29]. This supports a continuing role for 5-HT in subsequent cycles but does not exclude recruitment of additional mechanisms. Although the demographic and treatment factors predisposing to development of anticipatory nausea and vomiting are well defined (see [84], Table 1), the relationships between the outcome during cycle 1 and subsequent cycles is not and very few preclinical studies have attempted to mimic multicycle chemotherapy. Studies in the rat have shown that repeated doses of cisplatin exacerbate the initial gastric stasis and that the effect of granisetron in alleviating this delayed emptying reduced over doses of cisplatin [170]. Repeated doses of cisplatin in the rat (weekly for 5 weeks) also increased the number of enterochromaffin cells in the ileum [171] and caused an enteric neuropathy [169] which has also been reported to occur in mice with chronic oxaliplatin treatment [172]. The neuropathy differentially affects excitatory neurones leaving a relatively higher proportion of enteric inhibitory and nitrergic inhibitory neurones. Of particular interest is the observation that repeated doses of oxaliplatin in the rat upregulated spinal cord neuronal NOS (nitric oxide synthase) expression which has been linked to mechanical allodynia [103, 172], and this observation requires further study as similar changes in the NTS could have profound effects on emetic sensitivity. Overall these studies show that repeated doses of cytotoxic agents given to rodents over clinically relevant time periods can induce changes in the gut function and the related enteric nervous system that has major role in control of motility, secretion and blood flow [62]. In the same way that it was gradually realised that although mechanisms of acute and delayed chemotherapy differed and required different anti-emetic strategies, we may have to consider that the combination of mechanisms differs as chemotherapy progresses. For example, if some of the symptoms are due to the progressively changed gut motor function due to damage to excitatory neurones, then prokinetics working via facilitation of cholinergic neurones (e.g. motilin, $5\text{-}HT_4$ receptor agonists; [143]) will become progressively ineffective, but inhibitors on nitrergic neurones may be effective.

For most of these changes, we do not have any insights into how long the changes sustain, so it is quite possible that some of the processes initiated by the cytotoxic drug during cycle 1 are still in place during the next and subsequent cycles, and this together with the known plasticity of the emetic pathways [4] could contribute to the frequently observed reduction in anti-emetic efficacy. Although attention focuses on ototoxicity and sensory neuropathy as long-term toxicities of anticancer chemotherapy, additional consideration should be given to longer-term consequences for brain and gut function of the intense and prolonged activation of the emetic pathways.

2.10   Concluding Comments

In the 30 years since the first reports of the anti-emetic effects of a $5\text{-}HT_3$ receptor antagonist against cisplatin-induced emesis in the ferret [110], understanding of the mechanisms and pathways activated by cytotoxic drugs has transformed, facilitating advances in anti-emetic therapy most notably NK_1 receptor antagonists. Recent studies with "newer" $5\text{-}HT_3$ and NK_1 receptor antagonists (e.g. NEPA, [72]) discussed in other chapters in this book show considerable promise in approaching very high levels of complete control over multiple cycles. Whilst control of nausea has gradually improved, it still lags behind control of vomiting emphasising the need for studies in humans of the physiology of nausea and identification of clinically useful biomarkers for more objective assessment in clinical trials. The effects of anticancer chemotherapy agents on the body are clearly complex, but knowledge of the basic mechanisms by which the agents induce nausea and vomiting should allow the development of newer agents to optimise the anti-tumour effects whilst reducing the emetic liability, so acute and delayed CINV will no longer be an issue.

References

1. Alfieri AB, Cubeddu LX (1995) Treatment with para-chlorophenylalanine antagonises the emetic response and the serotonin-releasing actions of cisplatin in cancer patients. Br J Cancer 71(3):629–632
2. Allen ME, McKay C, Eaves DM, Hamilton D (1986) Naloxone enhances motion sickness: endorphins implicated. Aviat Space Environ Med 57(7):647–653
3. Andersen R, Krohg K (1976) Pain as a major cause of postoperative nausea. Can Anaesth Soc J 23(4):366–369

4. Andrews PLR, Davis CJ, Bingham S, Davidson HI, Hawthorn J, Maskell L (1990) The abdominal visceral innervation and the emetic reflex: pathways, pharmacology, and plasticity. Can J Physiol Pharmacol 68(2):325–345
5. Andrews PLR, Sanger GJ (2014) Nausea and the quest for the perfect anti-emetic. Eur J Pharmacol 722:108–121. doi:10.1016/j.ejphar.2013.09.072
6. Andrews PLR (1994) 5-HT$_3$ receptors and anti-emesis. In: King FD, Jones BJ, Sanger GJ (eds) 5-hydroxytryptamine-3 receptor antagonists. CRC Press, Boca Raton, pp 255–317
7. Andrews PLR, Davis CJ (1993) The mechanisms of emesis induced by anti-cancer therapies. In: Andres PLR, Sanger GJ (eds) Emesis and anti-cancer therapy. Chapman and Hall Medical, London, p 256
8. Andrews PLR, Rudd JA (2004) The role of tachykinins and the tachykinin receptor in nausea and emesis. In: Holzer P (ed) Handbook of experimental pharmacology, vol 164. Springer, Berlin, pp 359–440
9. Babaoglu MO, Bayar B, Aynacioglu AS, Kerb R, Abali H, Celik I, Bozkurt A (2005) Association of the ABCB1 3435C>T polymorphism with antiemetic efficacy of 5-hydroxytryptamine type 3 antagonists. Clin Pharmacol Ther 78(6):619–626. doi:10.1016/j.clpt.2005.08.015
10. Barcroft H, Swan HJC (1953) Sympathetic control of human blood vessels. Edward Arnold & Co., London
11. Barnes JM, Barnes NM, Costall B, Naylor RJ, Tattersall FD (1988) Reserpine, para-chlorophenylalanine and fenfluramine antagonise cisplatin-induced emesis in the ferret. Neuropharmacology 27(8):783–790
12. Barnes NM, Ge J, Jones WG, Naylor RJ, Rudd JA (1990) Cisplatin induced emesis: preliminary results indicative of changes in plasma levels of 5-hydroxytryptamine. Br J Cancer 62(5):862–864
13. Barreca T, Corsini G, Cataldi A, Garibaldi A, Cianciosi P, Rolandi E, Franceschini R (1996) Effect of the 5-HT$_3$ receptor antagonist ondansetron on plasma AVP secretion: a study in cancer patients. Biomed Pharmacother 50(10):512–514
14. Bearcroft CP, Andre EA, Farthing MJ (1997) In vivo effects of the 5-HT$_3$ antagonist alosetron on basal and cholera toxin-induced secretion in the human jejunum: a segmental perfusion study. Aliment Pharmacol Ther 11(6):1109–1114
15. Bermudez J, Boyle EA, Miner WD, Sanger GJ (1988) The anti-emetic potential of the 5-hydroxytryptamine3 receptor antagonist BRL 43694. Br J Cancer 58(5):644–650
16. Bertrand PP, Bertrand RL (2010) Serotonin release and uptake in the gastrointestinal tract. Auton Neurosci 153(1–2):47–57. doi:10.1016/j.autneu.2009.08.002
17. Beswick FW (1983) Chemical agents used in riot control and warfare. Hum Toxicol 2(2):247–256
18. Bhandari P, Gupta YK, Seth SD (1988) Effect of diethyldithiocarbamate on cisplatin induced emesis in dogs. Asia Pac J Pharmacol 3:247–250
19. Borison HL (1989) Area postrema: chemoreceptor circumventricular organ of the medulla oblongata. Prog Neurobiol 32(5):351–390
20. Borst P, Schinkel AH (2013) P-glycoprotein ABCB1: a major player in drug handling by mammals. J Clin Invest 123(10):4131–4133. doi:10.1172/JCI70430
21. Bouganim N, Dranitsaris G, Hopkins S, Vandermeer L, Godbout L, Dent S, Wheatley-Price P, Milano C, Clemons M (2012) Prospective validation of risk prediction indexes for acute and delayed chemotherapy-induced nausea and vomiting. Curr Oncol 19(6):e414–e421. doi:10.3747/co.19.1074
22. Brookes SJ, Spencer NJ, Costa M, Zagorodnyuk VP (2013) Extrinsic primary afferent signalling in the gut. Nat Rev Gastroenterol Hepatol 10(5):286–296. doi:10.1038/nrgastro.2013.29
23. Cannon DS, Best MR, Batson JD, Feldman M (1983) Taste familiarity and apomorphine-induced taste aversions in humans. Behav Res Ther 21(6):669–673
24. Caras SD, Soykan I, Beverly V, Lin Z, McCallum RW (1997) The effect of intravenous vasopressin on gastric myoelectrical activity in human subjects. Neurogastroenterol Motil 9(3):151–156

25. Castejon AM, Paez X, Hernandez L, Cubeddu LX (1999) Use of intravenous microdialysis to monitor changes in serotonin release and metabolism induced by cisplatin in cancer patients: comparative effects of granisetron and ondansetron. J Pharmacol Exp Ther 291(3):960–966

26. Christie DA, Tansey EM (2007) The discovery, use and impact of platinum salts as chemotherapy agents for cancer. Welcome Witn Twentieth Century Med 30:117

27. Ciarimboli G (2012) Membrane transporters as mediators of Cisplatin effects and side effects. Scientifica 2012:473829. doi:10.6064/2012/473829

28. Cubeddu LX (1992) Mechanisms by which cancer chemotherapeutic drugs induce emesis. Semin Oncol 19(6 Suppl 15):2–13

29. Cubeddu LX, Hoffmann IS (1993) Participation of serotonin on early and delayed emesis induced by initial and subsequent cycles of cisplatinum-based chemotherapy: effects of antiemetics. J Clin Pharmacol 33(8):691–697

30. Cubeddu LX, O'Connor DT, Hoffmann I, Parmer RJ (1995) Plasma chromogranin A marks emesis and serotonin release associated with dacarbazine and nitrogen mustard but not with cyclophosphamide-based chemotherapies. Br J Cancer 72(4):1033–1038

31. Cubeddu LX, O'Connor DT, Parmer RJ (1995) Plasma chromogranin A: a marker of serotonin release and of emesis associated with cisplatin chemotherapy. J Clin Oncol 13(3):681–687

32. Darmani NA, Crim JL, Janoyan JJ, Abad J, Ramirez J (2009) A re-evaluation of the neurotransmitter basis of chemotherapy-induced immediate and delayed vomiting: evidence from the least shrew. Brain Res 1248:40–58. doi:10.1016/j.brainres.2008.10.063

33. Darmani NA, McClanahan BA, Trinh C, Petrosino S, Valenti M, Di Marzo V (2005) Cisplatin increases brain 2-arachidonoylglycerol (2-AG) and concomitantly reduces intestinal 2-AG and anandamide levels in the least shrew. Neuropharmacology 49(4):502–513

34. Darmani NA, Ray AP (2009) Evidence for a re-evaluation of the neurochemical and anatomical bases of chemotherapy-induced vomiting. Chem Rev 109(7):3158–3199. doi:10.1021/cr900117p

35. Davis CJ, Harding RK, Leslie RA, Andrews PLR (1986) The organisation of vomiting as a protective reflex: a commentary on the first day's discussions. In: Davis CJ, Lake-Bakarr GV, Grahame-Smith DG (eds) Nausea and vomiting: mechanisms and treatment. Springer, Berlin, pp 65–75

36. De Jonghe BC, Horn CC (2008) Chemotherapy-induced pica and anorexia are reduced by common hepatic branch vagotomy in the rat. Am J Physiol Regul Integr Comp Physiol 294(3):R756–R765

37. De Jonghe BC, Horn CC (2009) Chemotherapy agent cisplatin induces 48-h Fos expression in the brain of a vomiting species, the house musk shrew (*Suncus murinus*). Am J Physiol Regul Integr Comp Physiol 296(4):R902–R911. doi:10.1152/ajpregu.90952.2008, 90952.2008 [pii]

38. Devinsky O, Frasca J, Pacia SV, Luciano DJ, Paraiso J, Doyle W (1995) Ictus emeticus: further evidence of nondominant temporal involvement. Neurology 45(6):1158–1160

39. Dey D, Abad J, Ray AP, Darmani NA (2010) Differential temporal changes in brain and gut substance P mRNA expression throughout the time-course of cisplatin-induced vomiting in the least shrew (*Cryptotis parva*). Brain Res 1310:103–112. doi:10.1016/j.brainres.2009.11.005

40. Di Maio M, Gallo C, Leighl NB, Piccirillo MC, Daniele G, Nuzzo F, Gridelli C, Gebbia V, Ciardiello F, De Placido S, Ceribelli A, Favaretto AG, de Matteis A, Feld R, Butts C, Bryce J, Signoriello S, Morabito A, Rocco G, Perrone F (2015) Symptomatic toxicities experienced during anticancer treatment: agreement between patient and physician reporting in three randomized trials. J Clin Oncol 33(8):910–915. doi:10.1200/JCO.2014.57.9334

41. du Bois A, Vach W, Wechsel U, Holy R, Schaefer W (1996) 5-Hydroxyindoleacetic acid (5-HIAA) and cortisol excretion as predictors of chemotherapy-induced emesis. Br J Cancer 74(7):1137–1140

42. Edwards CM, Carmichael J, Baylis PH, Harris AL (1989) Arginine vasopressin – a mediator of chemotherapy induced emesis? Br J Cancer 59(3):467–470

43. Eiseman JL, Beumer JH, Rigatti LH, Strychor S, Meyers K, Dienel S, Horn CC (2015) Plasma pharmacokinetics and tissue and brain distribution of cisplatin in musk shrews. Cancer Chemother Pharmacol 75(1):143–152. doi:10.1007/s00280-014-2623-5
44. Endo T, Sugawara J, Nemoto M, Minami M, Blower PR (1998) Effects of granisetron, a selective 5-HT$_3$ receptor antagonist, on ouabain-induced emesis in ferrets. Res Commun Mol Pathol Pharmacol 102(3):227–239
45. Erwald R, Wiechel KL, Strandell T (1976) Effect of vasopressin on regional splanchnic blood flows in conscious man. Acta Chir Scand 142(1):36–42
46. Eversmann T, Gottsmann M, Uhlich E, Ulbrecht G, von Werder K, Scriba PC (1978) Increased secretion of growth hormone, prolactin, antidiuretic hormone, and cortisol induced by the stress of motion sickness. Aviat Space Environ Med 49(1 Pt 1):53–57
47. Faas H, Feinle C, Enck P, Grundy D, Boesiger P (2001) Modulation of gastric motor activity by a centrally acting stimulus, circular vection, in humans. Am J Physiol Gastrointest Liver Physiol 280(5):G850–G857
48. Farmer AD, Al Omran Y, Aziz Q, Andrews PLR (2014) The role of the parasympathetic nervous system in visually induced motion sickness: systematic review and meta-analysis. Exp Brain Res 232(8):2665–2673. doi:10.1007/s00221-014-3964-3
49. Farmer AD, Ban VF, Coen SJ, Sanger GJ, Barker GJ, Gresty MA, Giampietro VP, Williams SC, Webb DL, Hellstrom PM, Andrews PLR, Aziz Q (2015) Visually induced nausea causes characteristic changes in cerebral, autonomic and endocrine function in humans. J Physiol 593(5):1183–1196. doi:10.1113/jphysiol.2014.284240
50. Feldman M, Samson WK, O'Dorisio TM (1988) Apomorphine-induced nausea in humans: release of vasopressin and pancreatic polypeptide. Gastroenterology 95(3):721–726
51. Fetting JH, Wilcox PM, Sheidler VR, Enterline JP, Donehower RC, Grochow LB (1985) Tastes associated with parenteral chemotherapy for breast cancer. Cancer Treat Rep 69(11):1249–1251
52. Finger TE, Kinnamon SC (2011) Taste isn't just for taste buds anymore. F1000 Biol Rep 3:20. doi:10.3410/B3-20
53. Fisher RD, Rentschler RE, Nelson JC, Godfrey TE, Wilbur DW (1982) Elevation of plasma antidiuretic hormones (ADH) associated with chemotherapy-induced emesis in man. Cancer Treat Rep 66(1):25–29
54. Forster ER, Palmer JL (1994) Comment: Ondansetron for treating nausea and vomiting in the poisoned patient. Ann Pharmacother 28(10):1203–1204
55. Foss JF, Yuan CS, Roizen MF, Goldberg LI (1998) Prevention of apomorphine- or cisplatin-induced emesis in the dog by a combination of methylnaltrexone and morphine. Cancer Chemother Pharmacol 42(4):287–291
56. Fredrikson M, Hursti T, Wik G (1995) Neural networks in chemotherapy-induced delayed nausea – a pilot-study using positron emission tomography. Oncol Rep 2(6):1001–1003
57. Fredrikson M, Hursti TJ, Steineck G, Furst CJ, Borjesson S, Peterson C (1994) Delayed chemotherapy-induced nausea is augmented by high levels of endogenous noradrenaline. Br J Cancer 70(4):642–645
58. Fukuda H, Koga T, Furukawa N, Nakamura E, Hatano M, Yanagihara M (2003) The site of the antiemetic action of NK$_1$ receptor antagonists. In: Donnerer J (ed) Antiemetic therapy. Karger, Basel, pp 33–77
59. Fukui H, Yamamoto M, Ando T, Sasaki S, Sato S (1993) Increase in serotonin levels in the dog ileum and blood by cisplatin as measured by microdialysis. Neuropharmacology 32(10):959–968
60. Fukui H, Yamamoto M, Sasaki S, Sato S (1993) Involvement of 5-HT$_3$ receptors and vagal afferents in copper sulfate- and cisplatin-induced emesis in monkeys. Eur J Pharmacol 249(1):13–18
61. Fukui H, Yamamoto M, Sato S (1992) Vagal afferent fibers and peripheral 5-HT$_3$ receptors mediate cisplatin-induced emesis in dogs. Jpn J Pharmacol 59(2):221–226
62. Furness JB (2012) The enteric nervous system and neurogastroenterology. Nat Rev Gastroenterol Hepatol 9(5):286–294. doi:10.1038/nrgastro.2012.32

63. Gal R (1975) Assessment of seasickness and its consequences by a method of peer evaluation. Aviat Space Environ Med 46(6):836–839
64. Gale DA, Blakemore SJ, Cook S, Kidwai S, Moore I, Moore GBT, Moore SE, Sanger GJ, Holbrook JD, Lui Y-L, Mailik N, Andrews PLR (2005) Modulation of gene expression in the glandular and non-glandular regions of the rat stomach after treatment with the anti-cancer drug cisplatin. Gastroenterology 128:A-545, Abstr T1762
65. Gilman A (1946) Therapeutic applications of chemical warfare agents. Fed Proc 5:285–292
66. Golding JF (2006) Motion sickness susceptibility. Auton Neurosci 129(1–2):67–76. doi:10.1016/j.autneu.2006.07.019
67. Gupta YK, Sharma SS (1996) Antiemetic activity of antioxidants against cisplatin-induced emesis in dogs. Environ Toxicol Pharmacol 1(3):179–184
68. Hagbom M, Istrate C, Engblom D, Karlsson T, Rodriguez-Diaz J, Buesa J, Taylor JA, Loitto VM, Magnusson KE, Ahlman H, Lundgren O, Svensson L (2011) Rotavirus stimulates release of serotonin (5-HT) from human enterochromaffin cells and activates brain structures involved in nausea and vomiting. PLoS Pathog 7(7), e1002115. doi:10.1371/journal.ppat.1002115
69. Harris AL (1982) Cytotoxic-therapy-induced vomiting is mediated via enkephalin pathways. Lancet 1(8274):714–716
70. Harris AL, Cantwell BMJ (1986) Mechanisms and treatments of cytotoxic-induced nausea and vomiting. In: Davis CJ, Lake-Bakaar GV, Grahame-Smith DG (eds) Nausea and vomiting: mechanisms and treatment. Springer, Berlin, pp 65–75
71. Hawthorn J, Ostler KJ, Andrews PLR (1988) The role of the abdominal visceral innervation and 5-hydroxytryptamine M-receptors in vomiting induced by the cytotoxic drugs cyclophosphamide and cis-platin in the ferret. Q J Exp Physiol 73(1):7–21
72. Hesketh PJ, Rossi G, Rizzi G, Palmas M, Alyasova A, Bondarenko I, Lisyanskaya A, Gralla RJ (2014) Efficacy and safety of NEPA, an oral combination of netupitant and palonosetron, for prevention of chemotherapy-induced nausea and vomiting following highly emetogenic chemotherapy: a randomized dose-ranging pivotal study. Ann Oncol 25(7):1340–1346. doi:10.1093/annonc/mdu110
73. Hesketh PJ, Van Belle S, Aapro M, Tattersall FD, Naylor RJ, Hargreaves R, Carides AD, Evans JK, Horgan KJ (2003) Differential involvement of neurotransmitters through the time course of cisplatin-induced emesis as revealed by therapy with specific receptor antagonists. Eur J Cancer 39(8):1074–1080
74. Higa GM, Auber ML, Altaha R, Piktel D, Kurian S, Hobbs G, Landreth K (2006) 5-Hydroxyindoleacetic acid and substance P profiles in patients receiving emetogenic chemotherapy. J Oncol Pharm Pract 12(4):201–209
75. Higa GM, Auber ML, Hobbs G (2012) Identification of a novel marker associated with risk for delayed chemotherapy-induced vomiting. Support Care Cancer 20(11):2803–2809. doi:10.1007/s00520-012-1402-2
76. Hirsch AT, Dzau VJ, Majzoub JA, Creager MA (1989) Vasopressin-mediated forearm vasodilation in normal humans. Evidence for a vascular vasopressin V_2 receptor. J Clin Invest 84(2):418–426. doi:10.1172/JCI114182
77. Horn CC, Ciucci M, Chaudhury A (2007) Brain Fos expression during 48 h after cisplatin treatment: neural pathways for acute and delayed visceral sickness. Auton Neurosci 132(1–2):44–51
78. Horn CC, De Jonghe BC, Matyas K, Norgren R (2009) Chemotherapy-induced kaolin intake is increased by lesion of the lateral parabrachial nucleus of the rat. Am J Physiol Regul Integr Comp Physiol 297(5):R1375–R1382. doi:10.1152/ajpregu.00284.2009
79. Horn CC, Kimball BA, Wang H, Kaus J, Dienel S, Nagy A, Gathright GR, Yates BJ, Andrews PLR (2013) Why can't rodents vomit? A comparative behavioral, anatomical, and physiological study. PLoS ONE 8(4), e60537. doi:10.1371/journal.pone.0060537
80. Horn CC, Richardson EJ, Andrews PLR, Friedman MI (2004) Differential effects on gastrointestinal and hepatic vagal afferent fibers in the rat by the anti-cancer agent cisplatin. Auton Neurosci 115(1–2):74–81

81. Hu DL, Zhu G, Mori F, Omoe K, Okada M, Wakabayashi K, Kaneko S, Shinagawa K, Nakane A (2007) Staphylococcal enterotoxin induces emesis through increasing serotonin release in intestine and it is downregulated by cannabinoid receptor 1. Cell Microbiol 9(9):2267–2277. doi:10.1111/j.1462-5822.2007.00957.x

82. Hursti TJ, Borjeson S, Hellstrom PM, Avall-Lundqvist E, Stock S, Steineck G, Peterson C (2005) Effect of chemotherapy on circulating gastrointestinal hormone levels in ovarian cancer patients: relationship to nausea and vomiting. Scand J Gastroenterol 40(6):654–661

83. Hursti TJ, Fredrikson M, Steineck G, Borjeson S, Furst CJ, Peterson C (1993) Endogenous cortisol exerts antiemetic effect similar to that of exogenous corticosteroids. Br J Cancer 68(1):112–114

84. Janelsins MC, Tejani MA, Kamen C, Peoples AR, Mustian KM, Morrow GR (2013) Current pharmacotherapy for chemotherapy-induced nausea and vomiting in cancer patients. Expert Opin Pharmacother 14(6):757–766. doi:10.1517/14656566.2013.776541

85. Jarve RK, Aggarwal SK (1997) Cisplatin-induced inhibition of the calcium-calmodulin complex, neuronal nitric oxide synthase activation and their role in stomach distention. Cancer Chemother Pharmacol 39(4):341–348. doi:10.1007/s002800050581

86. Jordan NS, Schauer PK, Schauer A, Nightingale C, Golub G, Martin RS, Williams HM (1985) The effect of administration rate on cisplatin-induced emesis. J Clin Oncol 3(4):559–561

87. Kiernan BD, Soykan I, Lin Z, Dale A, McCallum RW (1997) A new nausea model in humans produces mild nausea without electrogastrogram and vasopressin changes. Neurogastroenterol Motil 9(4):257–263

88. Kim J, Napadow V, Kuo B, Barbieri R (2011) A combined HRV-fMRI approach to assess cortical control of cardiovagal modulation by motion sickness. Conf Proc IEEE Eng Med Biol Soc 2011:2825–2828. doi:10.1109/IEMBS.2011.6090781

89. Kim MS, Chey WD, Owyang C, Hasler WL (1997) Role of plasma vasopressin as a mediator of nausea and gastric slow wave dysrhythmias in motion sickness. Am J Physiol 272(4 Pt 1):G853–G862

90. Kobrinsky NL, Pruden PB, Cheang MS, Levitt M, Bishop AJ, Tenenbein M (1988) Increased nausea and vomiting induced by naloxone in patients receiving cancer chemotherapy. Am J Pediatr Hematol Oncol 10(3):206–208

91. Koch KL (1997) A noxious trio: nausea, gastric dysrhythmias and vasopressin. Neurogastroenterol Motil 9(3):141–142

92. Kris MG, Gralla RJ, Clark RA, Tyson LB, O'Connell JP, Wertheim MS, Kelsen DP (1985) Incidence, course, and severity of delayed nausea and vomiting following the administration of high-dose cisplatin. J Clin Oncol 3(10):1379–1384

93. LaCount LT, Barbieri R, Park K, Kim J, Brown EN, Kuo B, Napadow V (2011) Static and dynamic autonomic response with increasing nausea perception. Aviat Space Environ Med 82(4):424–433

94. Ladabaum U, Koshy SS, Woods ML, Hooper FG, Owyang C, Hasler WL (1998) Differential symptomatic and electrogastrographic effects of distal and proximal human gastric distension. Am J Physiol 275(3 Pt 1):G418–G424

95. Landas S, Fischer J, Wilkin LD, Mitchell LD, Johnson AK, Turner JW, Theriac M, Moore KC (1985) Demonstration of regional blood-brain barrier permeability in human brain. Neurosci Lett 57(3):251–256

96. Leslie RA (1986) Comparative aspects of the area postrema: fine-structural considerations help to determine its function. Cell Mol Neurobiol 6(2):95–120

97. Lindstrom PA, Brizzee KR (1962) Relief of intractable vomiting from surgical lesions in the area postrema. J Neurosurg 19:228–236

98. Lumsden K, Holden WS (1969) The act of vomiting in man. Gut 10(3):173–179

99. Malik NM, Moore GB, Kaur R, Liu YL, Wood SL, Morrow RW, Sanger GJ, Andrews PLR (2008) Adaptive upregulation of gastric and hypothalamic ghrelin receptors and increased plasma ghrelin in a model of cancer chemotherapy-induced dyspepsia. Regul Pept 148(1–3):33–38. doi:10.1016/j.regpep.2008.03.005

100. Maolood N, Meister B (2009) Protein components of the blood-brain barrier (BBB) in the brainstem area postrema-nucleus tractus solitarius region. J Chem Neuroanat 37(3):182–195. doi:10.1016/j.jchemneu.2008.12.007
101. McWhinney SR, Goldberg RM, McLeod HL (2009) Platinum neurotoxicity pharmacogenetics. Mol Cancer Ther 8(1):10–16. doi:10.1158/1535-7163.MCT-08-0840
102. Miaskiewicz SL, Stricker EM, Verbalis JG (1989) Neurohypophyseal secretion in response to cholecystokinin but not meal-induced gastric distention in humans. J Clin Endocrinol Metab 68(4):837–843. doi:10.1210/jcem-68-4-837
103. Mihara Y, Egashira N, Sada H, Kawashiri T, Ushio S, Yano T, Ikesue H, Oishi R (2011) Involvement of spinal NR2B-containing NMDA receptors in oxaliplatin-induced mechanical allodynia in rats. Mol Pain 7:8. doi:10.1186/1744-8069-7-8
104. Miller AD, Rowley HA, Roberts TP, Kucharczyk J (1996) Human cortical activity during vestibular- and drug-induced nausea detected using MSI. Ann N Y Acad Sci 781:670–672
105. Miller AD, Rowley HA, Roberts TP, Kucharczyke J (1995) Activity of human cewrebral cortex during nausea recovery after ondansetron, as detected by magnetic source imaging. In: Serotonin and the scientific basis of anti-emetic therapy. Oxford Clinical Communications, Oxford, p 252
106. Miller CM, Wang BH, Moon SJ, Chen E, Wang H (2014) Neurenteric cyst of the area postrema. Case Rep Neurol Med 2014:718415. doi:10.1155/2014/718415
107. Minami M, Endo T, Hirafuji M, Hamaue N, Liu Y, Hiroshige T, Nemoto M, Saito H, Yoshioka M (2003) Pharmacological aspects of anticancer drug-induced emesis with emphasis on serotonin release and vagal nerve activity. Pharmacol Ther 99(2):149–165
108. Minami M, Endo T, Yokota H, Ogawa T, Nemoto M, Hamaue N, Hirafuji M, Yoshioka M, Nagahisa A, Andrews PLR (2001) Effects of CP-99, 994, a tachykinin NK(1) receptor antagonist, on abdominal afferent vagal activity in ferrets: evidence for involvement of NK(1) and 5-HT(3) receptors. Eur J Pharmacol 428(2):215–220
109. Minami M, Ogawa T, Endo T, Hamaue N, Hirafuji M, Yoshioka M, Blower PR, Andrews PLR (1997) Cyclophosphamide increases 5-hydroxytryptamine release from the isolated ileum of the rat. Res Commun Mol Pathol Pharmacol 97(1):13–24
110. Miner WD, Sanger GJ (1986) Inhibition of cisplatin-induced vomiting by selective 5-hydroxytryptamine M-receptor antagonism. Br J Pharmacol 88(3):497–499
111. Modlin IM, Kidd M, Pfragner R, Eick GN, Champaneria MC (2006) The functional characterization of normal and neoplastic human enterochromaffin cells. J Clin Endocrinol Metab 91(6):2340–2348. doi:10.1210/jc.2006-0110
112. Morrow GR (1984) Susceptibility to motion sickness and chemotherapy-induced side-effects. Lancet 1(8373):390–391
113. Morrow GR, Andrews PLR, Hickok JT, Stern R (2000) Vagal changes following cancer chemotherapy: implications for the development of nausea. Psychophysiology 37(3):378–384
114. Morrow GR, Angel C, Dubeshter B (1992) Autonomic changes during cancer chemotherapy induced nausea and emesis. Br J Cancer Suppl 19:S42–S45
115. Morrow GR, Hickok JT, Andrews PLR, Stern RM (2002) Reduction in serum cortisol after platinum based chemotherapy for cancer: a role for the HPA axis in treatment-related nausea? Psychophysiology 39(4):491–495
116. Morrow GR, Hickok JT, DuBeshter B, Lipshultz SE (1999) Changes in clinical measures of autonomic nervous system function related to cancer chemotherapy-induced nausea. J Auton Nerv Syst 78(1):57–63
117. Mowrey DB, Clayson DE (1982) Motion sickness, ginger, and psychophysics. Lancet 1(8273):655–657
118. Mutoh M, Imanishi H, Torii Y, Tamura M, Saito H, Matsuki N (1992) Cisplatin-induced emesis in *Suncus murinus*. Jpn J Pharmacol 58(3):321–324
119. Nalivaiko E, Rudd JA, So RHY (2015) Motion sickness, nausea and thermoregulation: the toxic hypothesis. Temperature 1:164–171
120. Napadow V, Sheehan J, Kim J, Dassatti A, Thurler AH, Surjanhata B, Vangel M, Makris N, Schaechter JD, Kuo B (2013) Brain white matter microstructure is associated with

susceptibility to motion-induced nausea. Neurogastroenterol Motil 25(5):448–450. doi:10.1111/nmo.12084, e303

121. Napadow V, Sheehan JD, Kim J, Lacount LT, Park K, Kaptchuk TJ, Rosen BR, Kuo B (2013) The brain circuitry underlying the temporal evolution of nausea in humans. Cereb Cortex 23(4):806–813. doi:10.1093/cercor/bhs073

122. Nussey SS, Hawthorn J, Page SR, Ang VT, Jenkins JS (1988) Responses of plasma oxytocin and arginine vasopressin to nausea induced by apomorphine and ipecacuanha. Clin Endocrinol (Oxf) 28(3):297–304

123. Oman CM (2012) Are evolutionary hypotheses for motion sickness "just-so" stories? J Vestib Res 22(2):117–127. doi:10.3233/VES-2011-0432

124. Page SR, Peterson DB, Crosby SR, Ang VT, White A, Jenkins JS, Nussey SS (1990) The responses of arginine vasopressin and adrenocorticotrophin to nausea induced by ipecacuanha. Clin Endocrinol (Oxf) 33(6):761–770

125. Percie du Sert N, Andrews PLR (2014) The ferret in nausea and vomiting research: lessons in translation of basic science to clinic. In: Biology and diseases of the ferret. Wiley, New Jersey, pp 735–778

126. Percie du Sert N, Rudd JA, Apfel CC, Andrews PLR (2011) Cisplatin-induced emesis: systematic review and meta-analysis of the ferret model and the effects of 5-HT(3) receptor antagonists. Cancer Chemother Pharmacol 67(3):667–686. doi:10.1007/s00280-010-1339-4

127. Percie du Sert N, Rudd JA, Moss R, Andrews PLR (2009) The delayed phase of cisplatin-induced emesis is mediated by the area postrema and not the abdominal visceral innervation in the ferret. Neurosci Lett 465(1):16–20. doi:10.1016/j.neulet.2009.08.075, S0304-3940(09)01181-1 [pii]

128. Perry MR, Rhee J, Smith WL (1994) Plasma levels of peptide YY correlate with cisplatin-induced emesis in dogs. J Pharm Pharmacol 46(7):553–557

129. Peyrot des Gachons C, Beauchamp GK, Stern RM, Koch KL, Breslin PA (2011) Bitter taste induces nausea. Curr Biol CB 21(7):R247–R248. doi:10.1016/j.cub.2011.02.028

130. Pi-Sunyer FX, Aronne LJ, Heshmati HM, Devin J, Rosenstock J (2006) Effect of rimonabant, a cannabinoid-1 receptor blocker, on weight and cardiometabolic risk factors in overweight or obese patients: RIO-North America: a randomized controlled trial. JAMA 295(7):761–775

131. Pivot X, Marghali N, Etienne MC, Bensadoun RJ, Thyss A, Otto J, Francois E, Renee N, Lagrange JL, Schneider M, Milano G (2000) A multivariate analysis for predicting cisplatin-induced delayed emesis. Oncol Rep 7(3):515–519

132. Popescu BF, Lennon VA, Parisi JE, Howe CL, Weigand SD, Cabrera-Gomez JA, Newell K, Mandler RN, Pittock SJ, Weinshenker BG, Lucchinetti CF (2011) Neuromyelitis optica unique area postrema lesions: nausea, vomiting, and pathogenic implications. Neurology 76(14):1229–1237. doi:10.1212/WNL.0b013e318214332c

133. Racke K, Reimann A, Schworer H, Kilbinger H (1996) Regulation of 5-HT release from enterochromaffin cells. Behav Brain Res 73(1–2):83–87

134. Raghupathi R, Duffield MD, Zelkas L, Meedeniya A, Brookes SJ, Sia TC, Wattchow DA, Spencer NJ, Keating DJ (2013) Identification of unique release kinetics of serotonin from guinea-pig and human enterochromaffin cells. J Physiol 591(Pt 23):5959–5975. doi:10.1113/jphysiol.2013.259796

135. Ratelade J, Bennett JL, Verkman AS (2011) Intravenous neuromyelitis optica autoantibody in mice targets aquaporin-4 in peripheral organs and area postrema. PLoS ONE 6(11), e27412. doi:10.1371/journal.pone.0027412

136. Rojas C, Raje M, Tsukamoto T, Slusher BS (2014) Molecular mechanisms of 5-HT(3) and NK(1) receptor antagonists in prevention of emesis. Eur J Pharmacol 722:26–37. doi:10.1016/j.ejphar.2013.08.049

137. Rowe JW, Shelton RL, Helderman JH, Vestal RE, Robertson GL (1979) Influence of the emetic reflex on vasopressin release in man. Kidney Int 16(6):729–735

138. Rudd JA, Andrews PLR (2004) Mechanisms of acute, delayed and anticipatory vomiting in cancer and cancer treatment. In: Hesketh P (ed) Management of nausea and vomiting in cancer and cancer treatment. Jones and Barlett Publishers, New York, pp 15–66

139. Rudd JA, Cheng CH, Naylor RJ (1998) Serotonin-independent model of cisplatin-induced emesis in the ferret. Jpn J Pharmacol 78(3):253–260
140. Rudd JA, Cheng CH, Naylor RJ, Ngan MP, Wai MK (1999) Modulation of emesis by fentanyl and opioid receptor antagonists in *Suncus murinus* (house musk shrew). Eur J Pharmacol 374(1):77–84
141. Rudd JA, Ngan MP, Wai MK (1998) 5-HT$_3$ receptors are not involved in conditioned taste aversions induced by 5-hydroxytryptamine, ipecacuanha or cisplatin. Eur J Pharmacol 352(2–3):143–149
142. Rudd JA, Tse JY, Wai MK (2000) Cisplatin-induced emesis in the cat: effect of granisetron and dexamethasone. Eur J Pharmacol 391(1-2):145–150
143. Sanger GJ, Broad J, Andrews PLR (2013) The relationship between gastric motility and nausea: gastric prokinetic agents as treatments. Eur J Pharmacol 715(1–3):10–14. doi:10.1016/j.ejphar.2013.06.031
144. Schaub N, Ng K, Kuo P, Aziz Q, Sifrim D (2014) Gastric and lower esophageal sphincter pressures during nausea: a study using visual motion-induced nausea and high-resolution manometry. Am J Physiol Gastrointest Liver Physiol 306(9):G741–G747. doi:10.1152/ajpgi.00412.2013
145. Schworer H, Racke K, Kilbinger H (1991) Cisplatin increases the release of 5-hydroxytryptamine (5-HT) from the isolated vascularly perfused small intestine of the guinea-pig: involvement of 5-HT$_3$ receptors. Naunyn Schmiedeberg's Arch Pharmacol 344(2):143–149
146. Sclocco R, Kinm J, Garcia RG, Sheenan JD, Beissner F, Bianchi AM, Cerutti S, Kuo B, Barbieri R, Napadow V (2014) Brain circuitry supporting multi-organ autonomic outflow in response to nausea. Cerebral Cortex. doi:10.1093/cercor/bhu172
147. Scott RH, Woods AJ, Lacey MJ, Fernando D, Crawford JH, Andrews PLR (1995) An electrophysiological investigation of the effects of cisplatin and the protective actions of dexamethasone on cultured dorsal root ganglion neurones from neonatal rats. Naunyn Schmiedeberg's Arch Pharmacol 352(3):247–255
148. Sem-Jacobsen CW (1968) Vegetative changes in response to electrical brain stimulation. Electroencephalogr Clin Neurophysiol 24(1):88
149. Shih V, Wan HS, Chan A (2009) Clinical predictors of chemotherapy-induced nausea and vomiting in breast cancer patients receiving adjuvant doxorubicin and cyclophosphamide. Ann Pharmacother 43(3):444–452. doi:10.1345/aph.1L437
150. Shinpo K, Hirai Y, Maezawa H, Totsuka Y, Funahashi M (2012) The role of area postrema neurons expressing H-channels in the induction mechanism of nausea and vomiting. Physiol Behav 107(1):98–103. doi:10.1016/j.physbeh.2012.06.002
151. Shoji A, Toda M, Suzuki K, Takahashi H, Takahashi K, Yoshiike Y, Ogura T, Watanuki Y, Nishiyama H, Odagiri S (1999) Insufficient effectiveness of 5-hydroxytryptamine-3 receptor antagonists due to oral morphine administration in patients with cisplatin-induced emesis. J Clin Oncol 17(6):1926–1930
152. Sipiora ML, Murtaugh MA, Gregoire MB, Duffy VB (2000) Bitter taste perception and severe vomiting in pregnancy. Physiol Behav 69(3):259–267
153. Soderpalm AH, Schuster A, de Wit H (2001) Antiemetic efficacy of smoked marijuana: subjective and behavioral effects on nausea induced by syrup of ipecac. Pharmacol Biochem Behav 69(3–4):343–350
154. Stern RM, Koch KL, Andrews PLR (2011) Nausea: mechanisms and management. Oxford University Press, New York
155. Stott JJR (1986) Mechanisms and treatment of motion illness. In: Davis CB, Lake-Bakaar GV, Grahame-Smith DG (eds) Nausea and vomiting: mechanisms and treatment. Springer, Berlin, pp 110–129
156. Stricker EM, McCann MJ, Flanagan LM, Verbalis JG (1988) Neurohypophyseal secretion and gastric function: biological correlates of nausea. In: Takagi H, Oomura Y, Ito M, Otsuka M (eds) Biowarning system in the brain, a Naito Foundation symposium. University of Tokyo Press, Tokyo

157. Sugino S, Hayase T, Higuchi M, Saito K, Moriya H, Kumeta Y, Kurosawa N, Namiki A, Janicki PK (2014) Association of mu-opioid receptor gene (OPRM1) haplotypes with postoperative nausea and vomiting. Exp Brain Res 232(8):2627–2635. doi:10.1007/s00221-014-3987-9

158. Sugino S, Janicki PK (2015) Pharmacogenetics of chemotherapy-induced nausea and vomiting. Pharmacogenomics 16(2):149–160. doi:10.2217/pgs.14.168

159. Takeda N, Hasegawa S, Morita M, Matsunaga T (1993) Pica in rats is analogous to emesis: an animal model in emesis research. Pharmacol Biochem Behav 45(4):817–821

160. Thomford NR, Sirinek KR (1975) Intravenous vasopressin in patients with portal hypertension: advantages of continuous infusion. J Surg Res 18(2):113–117

161. Thomson AJ, Williams RJP, Resolva S (1972) The chemistry of complexes related to cis-Pt(II)NH3)Cl2. An anti-tumour drug. Struct Bond (Springer, Berlin) 11:1–46

162. Torii Y, Mutoh M, Saito H, Matsuki N (1993) Involvement of free radicals in cisplatin-induced emesis in *Suncus murinus*. Eur J Pharmacol 248(2):131–135

163. Torii Y, Saito H, Matsuki N (1994) Induction of emesis in *Suncus murinus* by pyrogallol, a generator of free radicals. Br J Pharmacol 111(2):431–434

164. Treisman M (1977) Motion sickness: an evolutionary hypothesis. Science 197(4302): 493–495

165. Tremblay PB, Kaiser R, Sezer O, Rosler N, Schelenz C, Possinger K, Roots I, Brockmoller J (2003) Variations in the 5-hydroxytryptamine type 3B receptor gene as predictors of the efficacy of antiemetic treatment in cancer patients. J Clin Oncol 21(11):2147–2155

166. Tsuji D, Kim YI, Nakamichi H, Daimon T, Suwa K, Iwabe Y, Hayashi H, Inoue K, Yoshida M, Itoh K (2013) Association of ABCB1 polymorphisms with the antiemetic efficacy of granisetron plus dexamethasone in breast cancer patients. Drug Metab Pharmacokinet 28:299–304

167. Ueno S, Matsuki N, Saito H (1987) *Suncus murinus*: a new experimental model in emesis research. Life Sci 41(4):513–518

168. Ullah I, Subhan F, Rudd JA, Rauf K, Alam J, Shahid M, Sewell RD (2014) Attenuation of cisplatin-induced emetogenesis by standardized Bacopa monnieri extracts in the pigeon: behavioral and neurochemical correlations. Planta Med 80(17):1569–1579. doi:10.1055/s-0034-1383121

169. Vera G, Castillo M, Cabezos PA, Chiarlone A, Martin MI, Gori A, Pasquinelli G, Barbara G, Stanghellini V, Corinaldesi R, De Giorgio R, Abalo R (2011) Enteric neuropathy evoked by repeated cisplatin in the rat. Neurogastroenterol Motil 23(4):370–378. doi:10.1111/j.1365-2982.2011.01674.x, e162–373

170. Vera G, Lopez-Perez AE, Martinez-Villaluenga M, Cabezos PA, Abalo R (2014) X-ray analysis of the effect of the 5-HT₃ receptor antagonist granisetron on gastrointestinal motility in rats repeatedly treated with the antitumoral drug cisplatin. Exp Brain Res 232(8):2601–2612. doi:10.1007/s00221-014-3954-5

171. Vera Pasamontes G, Uranga JA, Martin Fontelles MI, Abalo R (2012) Histopathology of the severe effects induced by repeated cisplatin in rat tissues. Neurogastroenterol Motil 24(Suppl 2):49

172. Wafai L, Taher M, Jovanovska V, Bornstein JC, Dass CR, Nurgali K (2013) Effects of oxaliplatin on mouse myenteric neurons and colonic motility. Front Neurosci 7:30. doi:10.3389/fnins.2013.00030

173. Wang Y, Aggarwal SK, Painter CL (1999) Immunocytochemical and in situ hybridization studies of gastrin after cisplatin treatment. J Histochem Cytochem 47(8):1057–1062

174. Warr D (2014) Prognostic factors for chemotherapy induced nausea and vomiting. Eur J Pharmacol 722:192–196. doi:10.1016/j.ejphar.2013.10.015

175. Wicks D, Wright J, Rayment P, Spiller R (2005) Impact of bitter taste on gastric motility. Eur J Gastroenterol Hepatol 17(9):961–965

176. Wilder-Smith OH, Borgeat A, Chappuis P, Fathi M, Forni M (1993) Urinary serotonin metabolite excretion during cisplatin chemotherapy. Cancer 72(7):2239–2241

177. Willis CL, Garwood CJ, Ray DE (2007) A size selective vascular barrier in the rat area pos-trema formed by perivascular macrophages and the extracellular matrix. Neuroscience 150(2):498–509
178. Xu LH, Koch KL, Summy-Long J, Stern RM, Seaton JF, Harrison TS, Demers LM, Bingaman S (1993) Hypothalamic and gastric myoelectrical responses during vection-induced nausea in healthy Chinese subjects. Am J Physiol 265(4 Pt 1):E578–E584
179. Yu X, Yang J, Hou X, Zhang K, Qian W, Chen JD (2009) Cisplatin-induced gastric dysrhyth-mia and emesis in dogs and possible role of gastric electrical stimulation. Dig Dis Sci 54(5):922–927. doi:10.1007/s10620-008-0470-0
180. Zabara J, Chaffee RB Jr, Tansy MF (1972) Neuroinhibition in the regulation of emesis. Space Life Sci 3(3):282–292
181. Zoto T, Kilickap S, Yasar U, Celik I, Bozkurt A, Babaoglu MO (2015) Improved anti-emetic efficacy of 5-HT3 receptor antagonists in cancer patients with genetic polymorphisms of ABCB1 (MDR1) drug transporter. Basic Clin Pharmacol Toxicol 116(4):354–360. doi:10.1111/bcpt.12334
182. Zueva L, Rivera Y, Kucheryavykh L, Skatchkov SN, Eaton MJ, Sanabria P, Inyushin M (2014) Electron microscopy in rat brain slices reveals rapid accumulation of Cisplatin on ribosomes and other cellular components only in glia. Chemother Res Pract 2014:174039. doi:10.1155/2014/174039

Chapter 3
First-Generation 5-HT3 Receptor Antagonists

Roy Chen, Kathy Deng, and Harry Raftopoulos

3.1 Introduction

Chemotherapy-induced nausea and vomiting (CINV) is a significant side effect of cancer therapy and can lead to poor compliance with therapy, treatment delays, dehydration, hospitalization, and a marked decrement in patient quality of life. With appropriate CINV control, safe outpatient administration of chemotherapy can be accomplished with no change in patients' pre-therapy quality of life. Over the last 30 years, developments have improved in the control of CINV, including the advent of 5-hydroxytryptamine-3 (5-HT3) receptor antagonists which are an integral ingredient in regimens used today. With the variety of chemotherapy regimens today and the ongoing development of new combinations in addition to targeted therapy, there have been corresponding dynamic goals for control of not only CINV in general but in differentiating control of nausea over and above that of vomiting. In fact, current antiemetic therapy conceptually fulfills the true definition of "targeted therapy" as there is significant understanding of pathways involved in emesis as well as specific targeted antagonists to these pathways. This chapter will focus on the 5-HT3 pathway and the specific receptor antagonists to this pathway.

R. Chen, MD
Hematology-Oncology,
North Shore Hematology Oncology Associates,
East Setauket, NY, USA
e-mail: roybert318@gmail.com

K. Deng, MD
Hematology-Oncology, North Shore LIJ School of Medicine,
Hempstead, NY, USA

H. Raftopoulos, MD (✉)
Merck & Co., Rahway, NY, USA
e-mail: harry.raftopoulos@gmail.com

© Springer International Publishing Switzerland 2016
R.M. Navari (ed.), *Management of Chemotherapy-Induced Nausea and Vomiting: New Agents and New Uses of Current Agents*,
DOI 10.1007/978-3-319-27016-6_3

3.2 Physiology of CINV

The intrinsic emetogenicity of a given chemotherapeutic agent is the key determinant of the probability of clinical emesis, although chemotherapy dose, as well as patient factors such as female gender and young age may increase the probability of emesis [1]. Guideline groups divide chemotherapeutic agents into four emetogenic groups: high, moderate, low, and minimum [2] (Table 3.1). The clinical phases of emesis have been defined largely from observations using cisplatin where typically in the absence of antiemetics all patients will experience nausea and vomiting 1–2 h post administration. At 18–24 h the CINV abates, only to resurface and peak again at 48–72 h after the cisplatin administration [3]. As a result, acute emesis is defined as occurring within the

Table 3.1 Emetogenic potential of antineoplastic agents

Highly emetogenic (IV)	AC (doxorubicin or epirubicin with cyclophosphamide)	Dacarbazine	Ifosfamide >2 g/m^2 per dose
	Carmustine >250 mg/m^2	Doxorubicin >60 mg/m^2	Mechlorethamine
	Cisplatin	Epirubicin >90 mg/m^2	Streptozocin
	Cyclophosphamide >1,500 mg/m^2		
Moderately emetogenic (IV)	Aldesleukin >12–15 million IU/m^2	Clofarabine	Ifosfamide <2 g/m^2 per dose
	Amifostine >300 mg/m^2	Cyclophosphamide <1,500 mg/m^2	Interferon alfa >10 million IU/m^2
	Arsenic trioxide	Cytarabine >200 mg/m^2	Irinotecan
	Azacitidine	Dactinomycin	Melphalan
	Bendamustine	Daunorubicin	Methotrexate >250 mg/m^2
	Busulfan	Doxorubicin <60 mg/m^2	Oxaliplatin
	Carboplatin	Epirubicin <90 mg/m^2	Temozolomide
	Carmustine < 250 mg/m^2	Idarubicin	
Low emetic risk (IV)	Ado-trastuzumab emtansine	Etoposide	Paclitaxel
	Amifostine <300 mg	5-fluorouracil	Paclitaxel-albumin
	Aldesleukin <12 million IU/m^2	Floxuridine	Pemetrexed
	Brentuximab vedotin	Interferon alfa >5 <10 million IU/m^2	Pentostatin
	Cabazitaxel	Ixabepilone	Pralatrexate
	Carfilzomib	Methotrexate >50 mg/m^2 <250 mg/m^2	Romidepsin
	Cytarabine 100–200 mg/m^2	Mitomycin	Thiotepa
	Docetaxel	Mitoxantrone	Topotecan
	Doxorubicin (liposomal)	Omacetaxine	Ziv-aflibercept
	Eribulin		

Table 3.1 Continued

Minimal emetic risk (IV)	Alemtuzumab	Dexrazoxane	Pertuzumab
	Asparaginase	Fludarabine	Rituximab
	Bevacizumab	Interferon alfa <5 million IU/m²	Temsirolimus
	Bleomycin	Ipilimumab	Trastuzumab
	Bortezomib	Methotrexate <50 mg/m²	Valrubicin
	Cetuximab	Nelarabine	Vinblastine
	Cladribine	Ofatumumab	Vincristine
	Cytarabine <100 mg/m²	Panitumumab	Vincristine (liposomal)
	Decitabine	Pegaspargase	Vinorelbine
	Denileukin diftitox	Peginterferon	
Moderate to high emetic risk (oral)	Altretamine	Estramustine	Procarbazine
	Busulfan >4 mg/day	Etoposide	Temozolomide >75 mg/m²/day
	Crizotinib	Lomustine (single day)	Vismodegib
	Cyclophosphamide >100 mg/m²/day	Mitotane	
Minimal to low emetic risk (oral)	Axitinib	Gefitinib	Ruxolitinib
	Bexarotene	Hydroxyurea	Sorafenib
	Bosutinib	Imatinib	Sunitinib
	Busulfan <4 mg/day	Lapatinib	Temozolomide <75 mg/m²/day
	Cabozantinib	Lenalidomide	Thalidomide
	Capecitabine	Melphalan	Thioguanine
	Chlorambucil	Mercaptopurine	Topotecan
	Cyclophosphamide <100 mg/m²/day	Methotrexate	Trametinib
	Dasatinib	Nilotinib	Tretinoin
	Dabrafenib	Pazopanib	Vandetanib
	Erlotinib	Pomalidomide	Vemurafenib
	Everolimus	Ponatinib	Vorinostat
	Fludarabine	Regorafenib	

first 24 h and delayed after 24 h (usually up to 120 h) [2]. Other agents may also cause delayed emesis, although not usually with the same biphasic pattern as cisplatin.

Animal studies have defined significant neuroanatomic components of the emetic reflex. Initially, Thumas proposed a single vomiting center (dorsal vagal nucleus) in 1891 based on canine studies [4]; Wang and Borison further refined the concept to include a "sensor" area in the area postrema (often called the chemoreceptor trigger zone) and an "effector" area, the vomiting center, in the medulla [5]. More recent studies suggest two areas of afferent input in the dorsal vagal nucleus, the area postrema and the nucleus tractus solitarius, and rather than a discrete "vomiting center," several neuronal areas loosely organized to effect the emetic reflex, termed the "central pattern generator" [6].

The neurotransmitters involved in the emetic reflex related to chemotherapy are underpinned by 5-hydroxytryptamine (5-HT). Chemotherapy administration leads to local release of mediators by enterochromaffin cells in the proximal small intestine. These mediators include 5-HT, substance P, and cholecystokinin, which then bind to respective receptors (5-HT3, neurokinin-1, and cholecystokinin-1) located on terminal ends of abdominal vagal efferents [7]. This binding leads to a signal conducted by these vagal fibers which terminates in the nucleus tractus solitarius and leads to activation of the central pattern generator. The local release of 5-HT in the gastrointestinal tract and signal transduction by the vagal afferents is thought to be the chief mechanism whereby chemotherapeutic agents cause emesis [7]. Direct stimulation of the chemoreceptor trigger zone as described by Wang and Borison is a further mechanism, albeit thought to be a less important mechanism with CINV [8].

3.3 Development of First-Generation 5-HT3 Antagonists

In 1985, studies showed that high-dose metoclopramide (a dopamine-2 receptor antagonist) combined with dexamethasone provided meaningful protection from cisplatin-induced emesis at the expense of significant extrapyramidal side effects [9]. Curiously, at that time, results could not be replicated with other dopamine-2 receptor antagonists, suggesting the antiemetic effect was mediated by interaction with another neurotransmitter receptor. The 5-HT3 receptor emerged as a likely mediator of the antiemetic effect, and the pharmaceutical industry employed various strategies to develop selective 5-HT3 receptor antagonists. These included:

(a) Screening indole analogues, leading to the development of ondansetron [10]
(b) Structure-activity relationships around cocaine resulting in the development of dolasetron [11]
(c) Using serotonin as a basis, yielding tropisetron [12]
(d) Structure-activity relationships around tropisetron developed granisetron [13]

The structures of the four first-generation 5-HT3 antagonists are shown in Fig. 3.1 [14–17]. Since ondansetron and granisetron are the most used agents with dolasetron no longer indicated for CINV and tropisetron in limited use, a greater focus will be devoted to ondansetron and granisetron. The role of 5-HT3 receptor antagonists in postoperative nausea and vomiting is beyond the scope of this text.

3.3.1 Ondansetron

Ondansetron is an indole derivative, selective 5-HT3 receptor antagonist with weak affinity for other 5-HT receptors and dopamine receptors. Oral formulations are rapidly absorbed with an approximate 60 % bioavailability [18]; ondansetron is

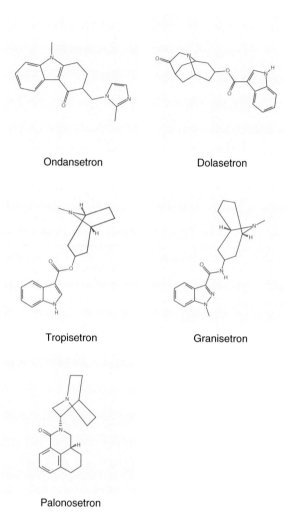

Ondansetron   Dolasetron

Tropisetron   Granisetron

Palonosetron

Fig. 3.1 Structures of the four first-generation 5-HT3 receptor antagonists and palonosetron

extensively metabolized primarily by hydroxylation of the indole ring with subsequent conjugation [19]. The elimination half-life is approximately 4 h (Table 3.2); metabolites are not significant contributors to activity. The elderly and patients with hepatic impairment show reduced clearance; however, this is not clinically meaningful [19].

Adverse events with ondansetron are largely confined to headache and constipation. An EKG study conducted in 2012 demonstrated significant QTc prolongation with a 32 mg dose of ondansetron prompting the FDA to limit the dose administered intravenously to 16 mg [20].

Table 3.2 5-HT3 receptor antagonist characteristics

5-HT3 receptor antagonist		Half-life (hours)	Oral bioavailability (%)	QTc prolongation
First generation	Ondansetron	4	59	Yes
	Dolasetron (hydrodolasetron)	7.3	76	Yes
	Tropisetron	8	60	Yes
	Granisetron	9	60	Yes
Second generation	Palonosetron	42	97	No

3.3.2 Dolasetron

Dolasetron is a selective 5-HT3 receptor antagonist derived after extensive chemical substitutions to the cocaine molecule. Dolasetron is rapidly metabolized to the active metabolite hydroxydolasetron, which is predominantly excreted in the urine and has an elimination half-life of 7.3 h (Table 3.2) [21]. Renal impairment increases the elimination time, but is once again not clinically relevant.

As with ondansetron, headache and constipation are the most significant adverse effects. QTc prolongation is also evident at higher doses, and in 2010, due to the QTc concerns, the approval for intravenous dolasetron in CINV was withdrawn.

3.3.3 Tropisetron

Tropisetron is another selective competitive antagonist of the 5-HT3 receptor, derived by chemical modification of serotonin (5-HT) and thus is also an indole derivative. Oral absorption is rapid with approximately 60 % bioavailability; metabolism is similar to ondansetron (hydroxylation followed by conjugation), with metabolites being inactive [22]. In most patients, the elimination half-life is approximately 8 h (Table 3.2), although in some poor metabolizers, the half-life may be up to 45 h [23]. Tropisetron is not available in the USA, but is used in the East and Australia.

3.3.4 Granisetron

Granisetron is a selective 5-HT3 receptor antagonist derived by making chemical alterations to tropisetron. Oral bioavailability is similar to other agents and metabolism is the primary means of elimination. The elimination half-life is approximately 9 h (Table 3.2), with no significant changes noted in elderly and those with renal or hepatic impairment [24]. In addition to the intravenous and oral formulations, a transdermal delivery system (patch) is available in the USA, delivering granisetron directly through intact skin by passive diffusion with levels peaking at 48 h and sustained for further 5 days. Adverse events once again include headache and constipation and reports of QTc prolongation.

3.4 Development of Palonosetron

Chemical strategies that examined conformational alterations in 5-HT3 receptor antagonists led to compounds with significantly increased affinity for the receptor and further alterations led to the development of palonosetron, deemed a second-generation 5-HT3 antagonist for its enhanced receptor binding affinity and prolonged half-life (approximately 42 h) (Table 3.2) [25]. The structure of palonosetron is shown in Fig. 3.1 [26]. In addition, distinguishing palonosetron from first-generation agents, it does not appear to have a meaningful effect on QTc [27]. Oral bioavailability is excellent at 97 % [28].

3.5 Clinical Studies

Over the last 30 years, numerous clinical studies have been conducted in the CINV space that have established the benefits of first-generation 5-HT3 receptor antagonists as well as have helped to refine dosing and steroid combinations. During the same period, standards and definitions as far as end points and study design have also evolved, such that initial studies had more variability in terms of measured end points and use of patient-reported outcomes. Currently, important definitions include the acute phase (0–24 h post emetogenic chemotherapy), delayed phase (24–120 h post), complete response (no emesis and no use of rescue medication), and complete control (no emesis and no more than minimal nausea) [1]. While not perfect, these standard definitions allow studies to be interpreted in context and determine whether any differences seen are meaningful. In addition, standardization has assisted in the development of meaningful guidelines to help translate clinical trial benefits to global benefits.

3.5.1 Initial Studies

3.5.1.1 Placebo-Controlled Studies

Two studies compared the efficacy of ondansetron and granisetron to placebo in preventing cisplatin-induced emesis. Cubeddu [29] randomized 28 chemotherapy-naive patients about to receive cisplatin to ondansetron or placebo as antiemetic prophylaxis. The control of emesis was significantly improved in the active treatment arm in terms of number of emetic episodes, time to emesis, and need for rescue medication. Cupissol [30] similarly randomized 28 chemotherapy-naive patients to receive granisetron or placebo with their first dose of cisplatin. Once again, the active therapy group had significant control of emesis – 13 of 14 granisetron patients had no acute nausea or vomiting whereas only 1 of 14 placebo patients was free of nausea or vomiting in the first 24 h. In patients receiving cyclophosphamide (at that time deemed a moderately emetogenic agent irrespective of the combination), Cubeddu randomized 20 patients to ondansetron or placebo [31] and predictably 70 % of ondansetron-treated patients experienced no emesis, compared to 0 % in the placebo arm. Two further studies in Japan used a placebo design to confirm the activity of ondansetron and tropisetron [32, 33]. The continued use of placebo controls was strongly discouraged except for studies involving low emetogenic risk agents, and further studies needed to compare new treatments with the best available existing therapy [34]. An individual patient data meta-analysis [35] reinforced the dismal outcome in terms of emesis control in placebo-treated patients.

3.5.1.2 Dose-Finding Studies

Principles of cancer supportive care, unlike primary therapy, dictate that the lowest effective dose of an agent can be used rather than the maximally tolerated dose: many initial studies sought to define optimal dosing of the first-generation 5-HT3 receptor antagonists. In patients receiving cisplatin, a double-blind trial of three different ondansetron doses (0.015, 0.15, and 0.30 mg/kg, each given three times 4 h apart) demonstrated the 0.15 mg/kg dose was superior to the lower dose, and no added improvement with the higher dose was noted [36]. Granisetron was also evaluated in patients receiving cisplatin in a double-blind study [37]. Doses evaluated were 2, 10, and 40 µg/kg with the 10 and 40 µg/kg doses being superior to the lower dose in terms of preventing cisplatin-induced CINV. There was no difference observed between the 10 and 40 µg/kg doses. A second study examined granisetron doses of 40 µg/kg or 160 µg/kg and found no differences in efficacy [38]. Similarly studies with tropisetron and dolasetron [39, 40] confirmed intermediate doses as effective in preventing cisplatin-induced CINV with no added benefit to dose escalation. Importantly, though, even at much higher doses than required for maximum efficacy, adverse events were seldom significantly increased.

3.5.1.3 Comparison Studies with Older Agents

Ondansetron (0.15-mg/kg × 3 doses) was compared with high-dose metoclopramide (2 mg/kg × 6 doses) in a single-blind trial in 307 patients receiving high-dose cisplatin [41]. Ondansetron was found to be superior to metoclopramide and produced fewer adverse events; in particular no extrapyramidal effects were noted with ondansetron. Similar findings were seen with two earlier smaller studies; however, the schedule of ondansetron administration was not standard (continuous infusion) [42, 43].

Granisetron trials provided clues that helped the understanding of the neurophysiology of emesis and the pharmacology of the antiemetics: granisetron alone was superior to either chlorpromazine or prochlorpromazine given together with dexamethasone for moderately emetogenic chemotherapy [44, 45]; yet when granisetron alone was compared to high-dose metoclopramide with dexamethasone for high-dose cisplatin, no differences in antiemetic control could be discerned [45, 46].

These observations validated the original findings by Gralla using metoclopramide and confirming the role of the 5-HT3 receptor in emesis. In addition clues about the utility of corticosteroids emerged.

3.5.2 The Role of Corticosteroids

Corticosteroids, in particular dexamethasone, have been used as antiemetics for CINV and have demonstrated efficacy, but no clear mechanism of action since their protective effects appear much sooner than conventional corticosteroid mechanism would allow. With the advent of 5-HT3 receptor antagonists, numerous studies examined the question of single-agent 5-HT3 receptor antagonist compared to corticosteroid combinations. The studies are summarized by Jantunen [47] and combining 11 studies in a meta-analysis demonstrated the odds ratio of acute vomiting to be 0.42, strongly in favor of the combination arms. The Italian Group for Antiemetic Research went further to define the optimal dosing of dexamethasone with 5-HT3 receptor antagonists both for highly emetogenic [48] and moderately emetogenic therapy [49].

3.5.3 First-Generation 5-HT3 Antagonists Compared

The first study to compare ondansetron to granisetron randomized 496 patients to receive either ondansetron 8 mg, ondansetron 32 mg, or granisetron 3 mg prior to cisplatin-based therapy [50]. No significant difference was seen between any of the groups related to emesis, nausea, or adverse events. Multiple other studies compared various doses or schedules of ondansetron with granisetron both as prophylaxis for highly emetogenic chemotherapy and for moderately emetogenic chemotherapy [51–56]. Other studies compared tropisetron [57, 58] as well as dolasetron [59–61]. Despite numerous studies, no significant differences emerged. Even large meta-analyses did not show any appreciable differences in clinical efficacy and adverse events [62, 63], although in the larger analysis, tropisetron was not as effective as granisetron [63].

3.5.4   Intravenous Compared to Oral Therapy

Oral forms of 5-HT3 receptor antagonists were developed shortly after the intravenous forms and theoretically provide more convenient dosing. The agents are well absorbed and undergo some first-pass metabolism although they are generally conserved; the bioavailability of oral ondansetron is 59 % [18], granisetron 60 % [64], tropisetron 60 % [22], and dolasetron (hydrodolasetron) 76 % [65].

Initial studies of oral 5-HT3 receptor antagonists examined ranges of oral doses and efficacy was significantly superior to historical placebo controls for ondansetron [66], dolasetron [67], and granisetron [68]. A direct systematic comparison of the same agent, comparing intravenous and oral forms in large randomized studies was only performed in a single study. The Ondansetron Acute Emesis Study Group randomized 530 patients to receive a single dose of either oral ondansetron 24 mg or intravenous ondansetron 8 mg together with dexamethasone prior to cisplatin therapy [69]. The acute (<24 h) complete response rates (no emesis and no rescue medication) were 85 % and 83 % for the oral and intravenous groups, respectively. Further randomized studies compared different formulations and agents: oral granisetron was compared to intravenous ondansetron prior to highly emetogenic therapy [70] and prior to moderately emetogenic therapy [71]; oral ondansetron was compared to intravenous granisetron prior to cisplatin therapy [72]. All three studies showed no difference in emesis control between randomized arms.

Oral 5-HT3 receptor antagonists allowed the opportunity to explore the use of these agents beyond the first day in an attempt to lessen delayed emesis. Some studies showed reduced delayed emesis with the use of 5-HT3 receptor antagonists beyond 24 h [73], while others failed to show any benefit [74]. A meta-analysis of ten randomized studies, including five that used dexamethasone in the delayed setting and five that did not, determined the reduction in emesis risk with longer treatment [75]. The absolute emesis risk reduction for monotherapy was 8.2 % (95 % CI, 3.0–13.4 %), whereas the reduction was only 2.6 % (95 % CI, −0.6–5.8 %) with the use of dexamethasone.

Oral therapy also allowed the evaluation of these agents in other oncology settings, particularly in preventing radiation-induced emesis. In patients receiving fractionated upper abdominal radiation, a randomized study of 260 patients demonstrated significant control of radiation-induced emesis with granisetron 2 mg daily compared with placebo [76]. Spitzer et al. [77] compared oral granisetron or ondansetron prior to total body irradiation to historical control patients. Emesis rates were significantly reduced in patients receiving either 5-HT3 receptor antagonist compared to the historical controls.

3.5.5   Summary of Characteristics of First-Generation 5-HT3 Receptor Antagonists

The four first-generation 5-HT3 receptor antagonists discussed here were derived from different processes but essentially exhibit more similarities than differences. These characteristics are listed below and are used as principles to formulate guideline recommendations for CINV prophylaxis:

(i)   They all contain an indole ring and are highly selective antagonists of the 5-HT3 receptor.
(ii) The elimination half-life is approximately 4–8 h.
(iii) Oral formulations are well absorbed with an approximate 60 % bioavailability and are equivalent to intravenous formulations.
(iv) The lowest effective dose has been determined.
(v)   Antiemetic efficacy is vastly superior to placebo for both highly and moderately emetogenic chemotherapy.
(vi) Antiemetic efficacy is superior to older antiemetics except for high-dose metoclopramide.
(vii) No significant differences in antiemetic efficacy are discernible between the four agents in individual studies.
(viii) Antiemetic efficacy is superior when combined with corticosteroids.
(ix) Side effects are largely confined to constipation and headache, with no appreciable increase in adverse events, even at escalated doses, although QTc prolongation has become a regulatory concern.

3.6   Palonosetron: A Second-Generation 5-HT3 Antagonist

Unlike the first-generation 5-HT3 antagonists, palonosetron is not based on an indole moiety; rather it contains a fused tricyclic ring and a quinuclidine moiety and has a half-life of approximately 40 h [28]. At the receptor level, it appears to bind to the 5-HT3 receptor more avidly than first-generation agents as well as exhibiting allosteric binding in contrast to the pure competitive binding seen with first-generation agents [78]. Further, it has been noted to cause receptor internalization [79], resulting in additional prolongation of duration of action. These unique properties are thought to account for some of the clinical efficacy differences seen in comparison to first-generation 5-HT3 receptor antagonists.

In the moderately emetogenic setting, palonosetron was compared to ondansetron [80] and dolasetron [81], respectively, in two double-blind randomized phase III trials. Both studies included three arms with only a single dose: palonosetron 0.25 mg and 0.75 mg and first-generation 5-HT3 receptor antagonist; no dexamethasone was administered as part of the protocol. Results from both studies demonstrated that a single dose of palonosetron (0.25 mg) was as effective as a single dose of a first-generation 5-HT3 receptor antagonist in preventing acute CINV and superior in preventing delayed CINV. In a randomized study conducted in the highly emetogenic setting, palonosetron was as effective as ondansetron and in a subset of patients also treated with dexamethasone appeared more effective [82].

Since the palonosetron registration studies were conducted without mandated corticosteroid therapy, the magnitude of benefit of palonosetron over the first-generation 5-HT3 receptor antagonists remained in question. A randomized study comparing palonosetron with dexamethasone to granisetron with dexamethasone in patients receiving highly or moderately emetogenic therapy helped to define the benefit [83]. There was no difference in the acute phase, but in the delayed phase, approximately 12 % more patients were emesis-free in the palonosetron arm as compared to the granisetron arm for both highly and moderately emetogenic therapy. Similar to first-generation 5-HT3 receptor antagonists, oral palonosetron has high bioavailability and similar efficacy to intravenous palonosetron with 0.5 mg being the preferred oral dose [84].

The improved efficacy observed with palonosetron has been attributed to the receptor-binding effects discussed above rather than the longer half-life, since administration of 5-HT3 receptor antagonists beyond day 1 results in negligible benefit in emesis control [75].

3.7 Novel Delivery Methods

Alternative routes of administration of first-generation 5-HT3 receptor antagonists have been explored, including subcutaneous, intramuscular, rectal, transdermal, and nasal/buccal sprays. In general, bioavailability of any route has been high with comparable efficacy where studied [85, 86]. Two delivery methods warrant further discussion: transdermal granisetron and polymer encapsulated slow-release granisetron.

3.7.1 Transdermal Granisetron

A transdermal formulation of granisetron is approved in the USA for the prevention of nausea and vomiting in patients receiving highly or moderately emetogenic chemotherapy. This granisetron transdermal delivery system is a 52 cm^2 patch containing 34.3 mg of granisetron, which is delivered transdermally as 3.1 mg/24 h and essentially achieves a similar exposure to that of a 2 mg oral dose providing continuous delivery of granisetron over 6 days [87]. A randomized, double-blind study included 641 patients receiving chemotherapy and demonstrated that the transdermal delivery system was non-inferior to oral granisetron [88]. Although balanced between treatment arms, the patient population studied was heterogeneous in terms of emetogenicity of chemotherapy (high or moderate), prior chemotherapy exposure and the use of corticosteroids. In addition, a strong limitation on the utility of this delivery system is the requirement to place patch 24 h before scheduled chemotherapy. Finally, since the benefit of first-generation 5-HT3 receptor antagonists beyond the first day of chemotherapy is limited [75], protracted delivery would appear to hold little advantage. Intuitively, such delivery systems may be more useful for preventing emesis from radiation or oral agents: no such studies have been conducted. Nevertheless, the transdermal system is approved in the USA and remains a potential choice for prevention of chemotherapy-induced nausea and vomiting.

3.7.2 Sustained-Release Subcutaneous Granisetron

APF530 is a subcutaneously administered polymeric formulation of granisetron that provides slow, controlled, and sustained release of granisetron [89]. APF530 comprises 2 % granisetron and a polymer that is designed to undergo controlled hydrolysis, imparting the drug release characteristics. In a phase 3 non-inferiority trial, the clinical efficacy of APF530 250 mg subcutaneously and 500 mg subcutaneously (containing granisetron 5 and 10 mg, respectively) was compared with 0.25 mg palonosetron intravenously in patients receiving moderately or highly emetogenic chemotherapy [90]. Patients were stratified according to emetogenicity of chemotherapy and received study drug together with appropriate placebo (subcutaneous saline for palonosetron group; intravenous saline for APF530 group). All patients received guideline-appropriate doses of dexamethasone. The study demonstrated non-inferiority of the 500 mg dose of APF530 compared with palonosetron in preventing CINV both in the acute and delayed setting. Since the classification of emetogenicity in the initial study design was based on the older Hesketh algorithm [91], a reanalysis of the study was undertaken, using the latest American Society of Clinical Oncology emetogenic classification [92]. The reanalysis confirmed the initial findings of non-inferiority of APF530 [93].

The observations from the single study of APF530 question the mechanism used to explain the superiority of palonosetron over first-generation 5-HT3 receptor antagonists: that receptor binding was more important than the extended half-life. A clear explanation to unify these observations will require further study.

3.8 Conclusion

First-generation 5-HT3 receptor antagonists dramatically altered the delivery of cytotoxic chemotherapy, changing intolerable regimens to tolerable ones, shifting many chemotherapy regimens to the ambulatory setting, and improving quality of life for many patients. Further understandings of the mechanisms of emesis and clinical trial observations have allowed refinements in their use; 5-HT3 receptor antagonists form the backbone of most antiemetic regimens. Improvements have also been seen with palonosetron and with newer agents such as neurokinin-1 receptor inhibitors; however, nausea remains a persistent problem and will require further refinements in the use of multiple agents, together with a better understanding of the mechanisms of chemotherapy-induced nausea to improve overall CINV control.

References

1. Markman M (2002) Progress in preventing chemotherapy-induced nausea and vomiting. Cleve Clin J Med 69:609–610, 612, 615–7
2. Roila F, Herrstedt J, Aapro M et al (2010) Guideline update for MASCC and ESMO in the prevention of chemotherapy- and radiotherapy-induced nausea and vomiting: results of the Perugia consensus conference. Ann Oncol 21(Suppl 5):v232–v243

3. Kris MG, Gralla RJ, Clark RA et al (1985) Incidence, course, and severity of delayed nausea and vomiting following the administration of high-dose cisplatin. J Clin Oncol 3:1379–1384

4. Thumas L (1891) Ueber das Brechcentrum und über die Wirkung einiger pharmakologischer Mittel auf dasselbe. Virchows Arch 123:44–69

5. Wang SC, Borison HL (1950) The vomiting center; a critical experimental analysis. Arch Neurol Psychiatry 63:928–941

6. Koga T, Fukuda H (1992) Neurons in the nucleus of the solitary tract mediating inputs from emetic vagal afferents and the area postrema to the pattern generator for the emetic act in dogs. Neurosci Res 14:166–179

7. Andrews PL, Davis CJ, Bingham S et al (1990) The abdominal visceral innervation and the emetic reflex: pathways, pharmacology, and plasticity. Can J Physiol Pharmacol 68:325–345

8. Leslie RA, Shah Y, Thejomayen M et al (1990) The neuropharmacology of emesis: the role of receptors in neuromodulation of nausea and vomiting. Can J Physiol Pharmacol 68:279–288

9. Kris MG, Gralla RJ, Tyson LB et al (1985) Improved control of cisplatin-induced emesis with high-dose metoclopramide and with combinations of metoclopramide, dexamethasone, and diphenhydramine. Results of consecutive trials in 255 patients. Cancer 55:527–534

10. Butler A, Hill JM, Ireland SJ et al (1988) Pharmacological properties of GR38032F, a novel antagonist at 5-HT3 receptors. Br J Pharmacol 94:397–412

11. Fozard JR, Mobarok Ali AT, Newgrosh G (1979) Blockade of serotonin receptors on autonomic neurones by (-)-cocaine and some related compounds. Eur J Pharmacol 59:195–210

12. Buchheit KH, Costall B, Engel G et al (1985) 5-Hydroxytryptamine receptor antagonism by metoclopramide and ICS 205–930 in the guinea-pig leads to enhancement of contractions of stomach muscle strips induced by electrical field stimulation and facilitation of gastric emptying in-vivo. J Pharm Pharmacol 37:664–667

13. Yan D, Schulte MK, Bloom KE et al (1999) Structural features of the ligand-binding domain of the serotonin 5-HT3 receptor. J Biol Chem 274:5537–5541

14. National Center for Biotechnology Information. PubChem Compound Database; CID = 4595. http://pubchem.ncbi.nlm.nih.gov/compound/ondansetron#section=Top. Accessed 11 Feb 2015

15. National Center for Biotechnology Information (2015) PubChem Compound Database; CID = 3148. http://pubchem.ncbi.nlm.nih.gov/compound/3148. Accessed 11 Feb 2015

16. National Center for Biotechnology Information (2015) PubChem Compound Database; CID = 656665. http://pubchem.ncbi.nlm.nih.gov/compound/tropisetron. Accessed 11 Feb 2015

17. National Center for Biotechnology Information (2015) PubChem Compound Database; CID = 5284566. http://pubchem.ncbi.nlm.nih.gov/compound/granisetron. Accessed 11 Feb 2015

18. Blackwell CP, Harding SM (1989) The clinical pharmacology of ondansetron. Eur J Cancer Clin Oncol 25(Suppl 1):S21–S24, discussion S25–7

19. Pritchard JF, Bryson JC, Kernodle AE et al (1992) Age and gender effects on ondansetron pharmacokinetics: evaluation of healthy aged volunteers. Clin Pharmacol Ther 51:51–55

20. Zuo P, Haberer LJ, Fang L et al (2014) Integration of modeling and simulation to support changes to ondansetron dosing following a randomized, double-blind, placebo-, and active-controlled thorough QT study. J Clin Pharmacol 54:1221–1229

21. Boxenbaum H, Gillespie T, Heck K et al (1992) Human dolasetron pharmacokinetics: I. Disposition following single-dose intravenous administration to normal male subjects. Biopharm Drug Dispos 13:693–701

22. Kees F, Farber L, Bucher M et al (2001) Pharmacokinetics of therapeutic doses of tropisetron in healthy volunteers. Br J Clin Pharmacol 52:705–707

23. Kim MK, Cho JY, Lim HS et al (2003) Effect of the CYP2D6 genotype on the pharmacokinetics of tropisetron in healthy Korean subjects. Eur J Clin Pharmacol 59:111–116

24. Carmichael J, Cantwell BM, Edwards CM et al (1989) A pharmacokinetic study of granisetron (BRL 43694A), a selective 5-HT3 receptor antagonist: correlation with anti-emetic response. Cancer Chemother Pharmacol 24:45–49

25. Clark RD, Miller AB, Berger J et al (1993) 2-(Quinuclidin-3-yl)pyrido[4,3-b]indol-1-ones and isoquinolin-1-ones. Potent conformationally restricted 5-HT3 receptor antagonists. J Med Chem 36:2645–2657

26. National Center for Biotechnology Information (2015) PubChem Compound Database; CID = 6337614. http://pubchem.ncbi.nlm.nih.gov/compound/Palonosetron. Accessed 11 Feb 2015
27. Yavas C, Dogan U, Yavas G et al (2012) Acute effect of palonosetron on electrocardiographic parameters in cancer patients: a prospective study. Support Care Cancer 20:2343–2347
28. Yang LP, Scott LJ (2009) Palonosetron: in the prevention of nausea and vomiting. Drugs 69:2257–2278
29. Cubeddu LX, Hoffmann IS, Fuenmayor NT et al (1990) Efficacy of ondansetron (GR 38032F) and the role of serotonin in cisplatin-induced nausea and vomiting. N Engl J Med 322:810–816
30. Cupissol DR, Serrou B, Caubel M (1990) The efficacy of granisetron as a prophylactic anti-emetic and intervention agent in high-dose cisplatin-induced emesis. Eur J Cancer 26(Suppl 1):S23–S27
31. Cubeddu LX, Hoffman IS, Fuenmayor NT et al (1990) Antagonism of serotonin S3 receptors with ondansetron prevents nausea and emesis induced by cyclophosphamide-containing chemotherapy regimens. J Clin Oncol 8:1721–1727
32. Ikeda M, Taguchi T, Ota K et al (1992) Evaluation of SN-307 (ondansetron), given intravenously in the treatment of nausea and vomiting caused by anticancer drugs including cisplatin – a placebo-controlled, double-blind comparative study. Gan To Kagaku Ryoho 19:2071–2084
33. Kondo M, Furue H, Taguchi T et al (1995) Clinical phase III study of tropisetron capsule in the treatment of nausea and vomiting induced by anti-cancer drug; a placebo-controlled, multi-center, double-blind comparative study. Gan To Kagaku Ryoho 22:1223–1234
34. McVie JG, de Bruijn KM (1992) Methodology of antiemetic trials. Drugs 43(Suppl 3):1–5
35. Kris MG, Cubeddu LX, Gralla RJ et al (1996) Are more antiemetic trials with a placebo necessary? Report of patient data from randomized trials of placebo antiemetics with cisplatin. Cancer 78:2193–2198
36. Grunberg SM, Lane M, Lester EP et al (1993) Randomized double-blind comparison of three dose levels of intravenous ondansetron in the prevention of cisplatin-induced emesis. Cancer Chemother Pharmacol 32:268–272
37. Riviere A (1994) Dose finding study of granisetron in patients receiving high-dose cisplatin chemotherapy. The Granisetron Study Group. Br J Cancer 69:967–971
38. Soukop M (1994) A dose-finding study of granisetron, a novel antiemetic, in patients receiving high-dose cisplatin. Granisetron Study Group. Support Care Cancer 2:177–183
39. Van Belle SJ, Stamatakis L, Bleiberg H et al (1994) Dose-finding study of tropisetron in cisplatin-induced nausea and vomiting. Ann Oncol 5:821–825
40. Kris MG, Grunberg SM, Gralla RJ et al (1994) Dose-ranging evaluation of the serotonin antagonist dolasetron mesylate in patients receiving high-dose cisplatin. J Clin Oncol 12:1045–1049
41. Hainsworth J, Harvey W, Pendergrass K et al (1991) A single-blind comparison of intravenous ondansetron, a selective serotonin antagonist, with intravenous metoclopramide in the prevention of nausea and vomiting associated with high-dose cisplatin chemotherapy. J Clin Oncol 9:721–728
42. De Mulder PH, Seynaeve C, Vermorken JB et al (1990) Ondansetron compared with high-dose metoclopramide in prophylaxis of acute and delayed cisplatin-induced nausea and vomiting. A multicenter, randomized, double-blind, crossover study. Ann Intern Med 113:834–840
43. Marty M, Pouillart P, Scholl S et al (1990) Comparison of the 5-hydroxytryptamine3 (serotonin) antagonist ondansetron (GR 38032F) with high-dose metoclopramide in the control of cisplatin-induced emesis. N Engl J Med 322:816–821
44. Warr D, Willan A, Fine S et al (1991) Superiority of granisetron to dexamethasone plus prochlorperazine in the prevention of chemotherapy-induced emesis. J Natl Cancer Inst 83:1169–1173
45. Marty M (1992) A comparison of granisetron as a single agent with conventional combination antiemetic therapies in the treatment of cytostatic-induced emesis. The Granisetron Study Group. Eur J Cancer 28A(Suppl 1):S12–S16

46. Warr D, Wilan A, Venner P et al (1992) A randomised, double-blind comparison of granisetron with high-dose metoclopramide, dexamethasone and diphenhydramine for cisplatin-induced emesis. An NCI Canada Clinical Trials Group Phase III Trial. Eur J Cancer 29A:33–36
47. Jantunen IT, Kataja VV, Muhonen TT (1997) An overview of randomised studies comparing 5-HT3 receptor antagonists to conventional anti-emetics in the prophylaxis of acute chemotherapy-induced vomiting. Eur J Cancer 33:66–74
48. Double-blind, dose-finding study of four intravenous doses of dexamethasone in the prevention of cisplatin-induced acute emesis. Italian Group for Antiemetic Research (1998) J Clin Oncol 16:2937–2942
49. Randomized, double-blind, dose-finding study of dexamethasone in preventing acute emesis induced by anthracyclines, carboplatin, or cyclophosphamide (2004) J Clin Oncol 22:725–729
50. Ruff P, Paska W, Goedhals L et al (1994) Ondansetron compared with granisetron in the prophylaxis of cisplatin-induced acute emesis: a multicentre double-blind, randomised, parallel-group study. The Ondansetron and Granisetron Emesis Study Group. Oncology 51:113–118
51. Noble A, Bremer K, Goedhals L et al (1994) A double-blind, randomised, crossover comparison of granisetron and ondansetron in 5-day fractionated chemotherapy: assessment of efficacy, safety and patient preference. The Granisetron Study Group. Eur J Cancer 30A:1083–1088
52. Ondansetron versus granisetron, both combined with dexamethasone, in the prevention of cisplatin-induced emesis. Italian Group of Antiemetic Research (1995) Ann Oncol 6:805–810
53. Bonneterre J, Hecquet B (1995) Granisetron (IV) compared with ondansetron (IV plus oral) in the prevention of nausea and vomiting induced by moderately-emetogenic chemotherapy. A cross-over study. Bull Cancer 82:1038–1043
54. Navari R, Gandara D, Hesketh P et al (1995) Comparative clinical trial of granisetron and ondansetron in the prophylaxis of cisplatin-induced emesis. The Granisetron Study Group. J Clin Oncol 13:1242–1248
55. Stewart A, McQuade B, Cronje JD et al (1995) Ondansetron compared with granisetron in the prophylaxis of cyclophosphamide-induced emesis in out-patients: a multicentre, double-blind, double-dummy, randomised, parallel-group study. Emesis Study Group for Ondansetron and Granisetron in Breast Cancer Patients. Oncology 52:202–210
56. Martoni A, Angelelli B, Guaraldi M et al (1996) An open randomised cross-over study on granisetron versus ondansetron in the prevention of acute emesis induced by moderate dose cisplatin-containing regimens. Eur J Cancer 32A:82–85
57. Chua DT, Sham JS, Kwong DL et al (2000) Comparative efficacy of three 5-HT3 antagonists (granisetron, ondansetron, and tropisetron) plus dexamethasone for the prevention of cisplatin-induced acute emesis: a randomized crossover study. Am J Clin Oncol 23:185–191
58. Oge A, Alkis N, Oge O et al (2000) Comparison of granisetron, ondansetron and tropisetron for control of vomiting and nausea induced by cisplatin. J Chemother 12:105–108
59. Audhuy B, Cappelaere P, Martin M et al (1996) A double-blind, randomised comparison of the anti-emetic efficacy of two intravenous doses of dolasetron mesylate and granisetron in patients receiving high dose cisplatin chemotherapy. Eur J Cancer 32A:807–813
60. Fauser AA, Duclos B, Chemaissani A et al (1996) Therapeutic equivalence of single oral doses of dolasetron mesylate and multiple doses of ondansetron for the prevention of emesis after moderately emetogenic chemotherapy. European Dolasetron Comparative Study Group. Eur J Cancer 32A:1523–1529
61. Lofters WS, Pater JL, Zee B et al (1997) Phase III double-blind comparison of dolasetron mesylate and ondansetron and an evaluation of the additive role of dexamethasone in the prevention of acute and delayed nausea and vomiting due to moderately emetogenic chemotherapy. J Clin Oncol 15:2966–2973
62. Hesketh PJ (2000) Comparative review of 5-HT3 receptor antagonists in the treatment of acute chemotherapy-induced nausea and vomiting. Cancer Investig 18:163–173
63. Jordan K, Hinke A, Grothey A et al (2007) A meta-analysis comparing the efficacy of four 5-HT3-receptor antagonists for acute chemotherapy-induced emesis. Support Care Cancer 15:1023–1033

64. Clarke SE, Austin NE, Bloomer JC et al (1994) Metabolism and disposition of 14C-granisetron in rat, dog and man after intravenous and oral dosing. Xenobiotica 24:1119–1131
65. Dimmitt DC, Choo YS, Martin LA et al (1999) Intravenous pharmacokinetics and absolute oral bioavailability of dolasetron in healthy volunteers: part 1. Biopharm Drug Dispos 20:29–39
66. Needles B, Miranda E, Garcia Rodriguez FM et al (1999) A multicenter, double-blind, randomized comparison of oral ondansetron 8 mg b.i.d., 24 mg q.d., and 32 mg q.d. in the prevention of nausea and vomiting associated with highly emetogenic chemotherapy. S3AA3012 Study Group. Support Care Cancer 7:347–353
67. Rubenstein EB, Gralla RJ, Hainsworth JD et al (1997) Randomized, double blind, dose-response trial across four oral doses of dolasetron for the prevention of acute emesis after moderately emetogenic chemotherapy. Oral Dolasetron Dose-Response Study Group. Cancer 79:1216–1224
68. Bleiberg HH, Spielmann M, Falkson G et al (1995) Antiemetic treatment with oral granisetron in patients receiving moderately emetogenic chemotherapy: a dose-ranging study. Clin Ther 17:38–51
69. Krzakowski M, Graham E, Goedhals L et al (1998) A multicenter, double-blind comparison of i.v. and oral administration of ondansetron plus dexamethasone for acute cisplatin-induced emesis. Ondansetron Acute Emesis Study Group. Anticancer Drugs 9:593–598
70. Gralla RJ, Navari RM, Hesketh PJ et al (1998) Single-dose oral granisetron has equivalent antiemetic efficacy to intravenous ondansetron for highly emetogenic cisplatin-based chemotherapy. J Clin Oncol 16:1568–1573
71. Perez EA, Hesketh P, Sandbach J et al (1998) Comparison of single-dose oral granisetron versus intravenous ondansetron in the prevention of nausea and vomiting induced by moderately emetogenic chemotherapy: a multicenter, double-blind, randomized parallel study. J Clin Oncol 16:754–760
72. Spector JI, Lester EP, Chevlen EM et al (1998) A comparison of oral ondansetron and intravenous granisetron for the prevention of nausea and emesis associated with cisplatin-based chemotherapy. Oncologist 3:432–438
73. Navari RM, Madajewicz S, Anderson N et al (1995) Oral ondansetron for the control of cisplatin-induced delayed emesis: a large, multicenter, double-blind, randomized comparative trial of ondansetron versus placebo. J Clin Oncol 13:2408–2416
74. Olver I, Paska W, Depierre A et al (1996) A multicentre, double-blind study comparing placebo, ondansetron and ondansetron plus dexamethasone for the control of cisplatin-induced delayed emesis. Ondansetron Delayed Emesis Study Group. Ann Oncol 7:945–952
75. Geling O, Eichler HG (2005) Should 5-hydroxytryptamine-3 receptor antagonists be administered beyond 24 hours after chemotherapy to prevent delayed emesis? Systematic re-evaluation of clinical evidence and drug cost implications. J Clin Oncol 23:1289–1294
76. Lanciano R, Sherman DM, Michalski J et al (2001) The efficacy and safety of once-daily Kytril (granisetron hydrochloride) tablets in the prophylaxis of nausea and emesis following fractionated upper abdominal radiotherapy. Cancer Invest 19:763–772
77. Spitzer TR, Friedman CJ, Bushnell W et al (2000) Double-blind, randomized, parallel-group study on the efficacy and safety of oral granisetron and oral ondansetron in the prophylaxis of nausea and vomiting in patients receiving hyperfractionated total body irradiation. Bone Marrow Transplant 26:203–210
78. Rojas C, Stathis M, Thomas AG et al (2008) Palonosetron exhibits unique molecular interactions with the 5-HT3 receptor. Anesth Analg 107:469–478
79. Rojas C, Thomas AG, Alt J et al (2010) Palonosetron triggers 5-HT(3) receptor internalization and causes prolonged inhibition of receptor function. Eur J Pharmacol 626:193–199
80. Gralla R, Lichinitser M, Van Der Vegt S et al (2003) Palonosetron improves prevention of chemotherapy-induced nausea and vomiting following moderately emetogenic chemotherapy: results of a double-blind randomized phase III trial comparing single doses of palonosetron with ondansetron. Ann Oncol 14:1570–1577

81. Eisenberg P, Figueroa-Vadillo J, Zamora R et al (2003) Improved prevention of moderately emetogenic chemotherapy-induced nausea and vomiting with palonosetron, a pharmacologically novel 5-HT3 receptor antagonist: results of a phase III, single-dose trial versus dolasetron. Cancer 98:2473–2482

82. Aapro MS, Grunberg SM, Manikhas GM et al (2006) A phase III, double-blind, randomized trial of palonosetron compared with ondansetron in preventing chemotherapy-induced nausea and vomiting following highly emetogenic chemotherapy. Ann Oncol 17:1441–1449

83. Saito M, Aogi K, Sekine I et al (2009) Palonosetron plus dexamethasone versus granisetron plus dexamethasone for prevention of nausea and vomiting during chemotherapy: a double-blind, double-dummy, randomised, comparative phase III trial. Lancet Oncol 10:115–124

84. Boccia R, Grunberg S, Franco-Gonzales E et al (2013) Efficacy of oral palonosetron compared to intravenous palonosetron for the prevention of chemotherapy-induced nausea and vomiting associated with moderately emetogenic chemotherapy: a phase 3 trial. Support Care Cancer 21:1453–1460

85. Gurpide A, Sadaba B, Martin-Algarra S et al (2007) Randomized crossover pharmacokinetic evaluation of subcutaneous versus intravenous granisetron in cancer patients treated with platinum-based chemotherapy. Oncologist 12:1151–1155

86. Roila F, Del Favero A (1995) Ondansetron clinical pharmacokinetics. Clin Pharmacokinet 29:95–109

87. Howell J, Smeets J, Drenth HJ et al (2009) Pharmacokinetics of a granisetron transdermal system for the treatment of chemotherapy-induced nausea and vomiting. J Oncol Pharm Pract 15:223–231

88. Boccia RV, Gordan LN, Clark G et al (2011) Efficacy and tolerability of transdermal granisetron for the control of chemotherapy-induced nausea and vomiting associated with moderately and highly emetogenic multi-day chemotherapy: a randomized, double-blind, phase III study. Support Care Cancer 19:1609–1617

89. Heller J, Barr J (2005) Biochronomer technology. Expert Opin Drug Deliv 2:169–183

90. Raftopoulos H, Cooper W, O'Boyle E et al (2015) Comparison of an extended-release formulation of granisetron (APF530) versus palonosetron for the prevention of chemotherapy-induced nausea and vomiting associated with moderately or highly emetogenic chemotherapy: results of a prospective, randomized, double-blind, noninferiority phase 3 trial. Support Care Cancer 23:723–732

91. Hesketh PJ, Kris MG, Grunberg SM et al (1997) Proposal for classifying the acute emetogenicity of cancer chemotherapy. J Clin Oncol 15:103–109

92. Basch E, Prestrud AA, Hesketh PJ et al (2011) Antiemetics: American Society of Clinical Oncology clinical practice guideline update. J Clin Oncol 29:4189–4198

93. Raftopoulos H, Boccia RV, Cooper W et al (2014) A prospective, randomized, double-blind phase 3 trial of extended-release granisetron (APF530) versus palonosetron (PALO) for preventing chemotherapy-induced nausea and vomiting (CINV) associated with moderately (MEC) or highly (HEC) emetogenic chemotherapy: does a reanalysis using newer ASCO emetogenicity criteria affect study conclusions? ASCO Meet Abstr 32:9648

Chapter 4
Palonosetron

Lee Schwartzberg

With the recognition that the 5-hydroxytryptamine receptor was important in mediating cisplatin-induced emesis, work at several pharmaceutical companies focused on creating drugs that interfered with serotonin binding utilizing a variety of medicinal chemistry strategies. The first-generation 5-hydroxytryptamine receptor antagonists (5-HT$_3$ RAs) ondansetron, granisetron, tropisetron, and dolasetron were structurally similar and showed activity in preventing chemotherapy-induced nausea and vomiting. However, complete response during the acute phase after cisplatin was achieved in only 50–70 % of patients and was substantially less effective in the delayed phase for control of both emesis and nausea. The first-generation 5-HT$_3$ RAs do not improve control of delayed CINV over dexamethasone alone [1], nor does prolonged administration provide much additional benefit [2]. In addition, the first-generation 5-HT$_3$ RAs were therapeutically equivalent with several large trials comparing these drugs to one another demonstrating similar efficacy [3, 4]. A plateau in 5-HT$_3$ RA activity had been reached. Efforts persisted to find potentially more active agents based on the understanding of the central importance of this specific serotonin receptor in ameliorating chemotherapy-induced emesis.

4.1 Development of Palonosetron

In 1993 researchers at Syntex Research in Palo Alto, California, created a new class of 5-HT$_3$ RAs [5] by making various substitutions to the chemical structure of the first-generation 5-HT$_3$ RAs and exploring their interactions with the 5-HT$_3$ receptor.

L. Schwartzberg, MD, FACP
Division of Hematology/Oncology, Department of Medicine,
University of Tennessee Health Science Center, Memphis, TN, USA
e-mail: lschwartzberg@westclinic.com

© Springer International Publishing Switzerland 2016
R.M. Navari (ed.), *Management of Chemotherapy-Induced Nausea
and Vomiting: New Agents and New Uses of Current Agents*,
DOI 10.1007/978-3-319-27016-6_4

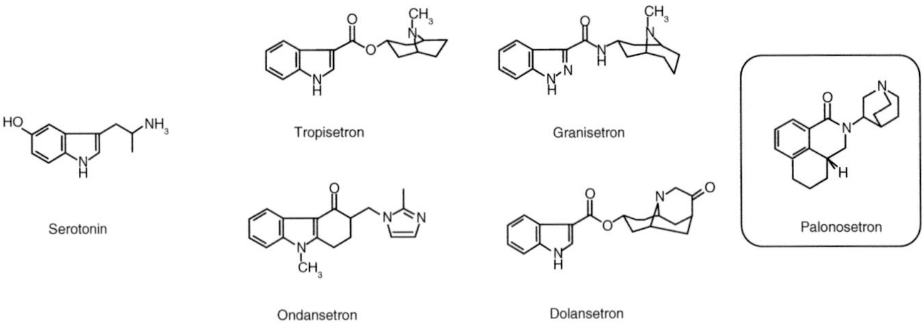

Fig. 4.1 Chemical structure of 5-HT$_3$ receptor antagonists

The highest-affinity compound, consisting chemically of a conformationally restrained alkano-bridged quinolone, was termed palonosetron, named for the place of discovery. Most 5-HT$_3$ RAs incorporate a three substituted indole resembling serotonin, whereas palonosetron is a fixed tricyclic ring attached to an isoquinolone moiety yielding a substantially different chemical structure (Fig. 4.1).

Palonosetron displays several pharmacologic characteristics which differ from other first-generation 5-HT$_3$ RAs which may account for its clinical distinction. The binding affinity of palonosetron is 2,500-fold higher than that of serotonin [6]. It has a much higher affinity constant (PK$_1$ = 10.45) for the 5-HT$_3$ receptor than the first-generation agents which are at least tenfold lower [7, 8]. The plasma half-life of palonosetron is approximately 40 h, while the other first-generation 5-HT$_3$ receptor antagonist's half-life ranges from 5 to 12 h [9, 10]. It is excreted predominantly in the urine, with much of the parent compound excreted unmetabolized in contrast to ondansetron which is heavily metabolized [11].

In addition to these pharmacokinetic differences, palonosetron displays qualitative and quantitative biologic and physiologic differences from the other agents. Using tritium-labeled palonosetron, granisetron, and ondansetron, Rojas et al. [12] demonstrated that palonosetron acts as an allosteric antagonist with positive cooperativity. Palonosetron binds to additional sites in the 5-HT$_3$ receptor besides the ones that bind ondansetron or granisetron inducing a conformational change. Additionally, receptor-associated palonosetron is retained in cell culture experiments after prolonged dilution and washings suggesting that the bound palonosetron is internalized [13].

Support for a functional consequence of allosteric binding comes from experiments demonstrating that granisetron and ondansetron as well as palonosetron inhibit calcium iron influx through the serotonin receptor. Calcium influx is the normal physiologic effect representative of serotonin receptor-triggered signaling when cells are preincubated with granisetron or ondansetron and then rinsed multiple times to remove any trace of the drug, they recover the ability to respond to serotonin. In contrast, when palonosetron is preincubated and cells are washed, interference with calcium influx is retained. These effects were not seen when ondansetron was used as the binding agent to the 5-HT$_3$ receptor and was minimal with granisetron. Long-term calcium influx inhibition may represent one reason why palonosetron is a more effective drug than the first-generation agents.

In further experiments, the same group demonstrated conclusive evidence of receptor internalization when cells were exposed to palonosetron but minimal internalization with granisetron and none with ondansetron [14]. The palonosetron-receptor complex remains internalized for at least 25 h after exposure to palonosetron, indicating that it interferes with receptor exocytosis, in contrast to serotonin where exocytosis and renewal of the cell membrane-associated receptor occur [15]. Overall, the palonosetron-5-HT_3 interaction leads to reduced receptor density at the cell surface and may be an additional explanation for the prolonged inhibition of receptor function.

An alternative hypothesis to explain the prolonged effect of palonosetron was proposed by another group of investigators who showed that palonosetron induced a long-term inhibition of the number of available 5-HT_3 receptor-binding sites due to slow disassociation from the receptor [16]. Palonosetron did not actually reduce cell surface expression of 5-HT_3 receptors and did not affect the rate of receptor endocytosis in these series of experiments. The investigators proposed that palonosetron works by pseudo-irreversible interactions with the 5-HT_3 receptors rather than receptor-ligand internalization.

Cross talk between NK1 and 5-HT_3 receptor signaling pathways has been reported by several different groups of investigators [17–19]. NK1 antagonists block vagal afferent activation by substance P, and 5-HT_3 receptor antagonists block vagal afferent activation by serotonin. This cross talk raises the possibility that palonosetron's unique efficacy as a 5-HT_3 receptor antagonist may be in part due to differential inhibition of the cross talk. In both in vitro and in vivo experiments, palonosetron inhibited NK1 receptor activation from substance P, a potent NK1 agonist [13]. This inhibition was dose dependent and was not seen in parallel experiments with granisetron or ondansetron. Taken together, palonosetron is a structurally unique, pharmacologically distinct agent with various different properties from the first-generation 5-HT_3 RAs which underlie its clinical differentiation (Table 4.1).

Palonosetron's interaction with NK1 was further evaluated experimentally using the potent NK1 antagonist netupitant [20]. Palonosetron exhibited a synergistic effect on inhibition of the substance P response in the presence of netupitant. The effect occurred using concentrations of each receptor antagonist below the threshold of inhibition of the substance P response and also concentrations where maximal inhibition of the substance P response was observed suggesting that in vivo the effect was clinically relevant.

Table 4.1 Summary of comparison among palonosetron, ondansetron, and granisetron

	Palonosetron	Ondansetron	Granisetron
Plasma half-life (h)	>40	5–6	12
Binding affinity (pK_i)	10.45	8.19	8.91
Positive cooperativity	Yes	No	No
Inhibition of receptor function	Long lasting	Short lasting	Short lasting
Receptor internalization	Yes	No	No
Inhibition of 5-HT_3/NK_1 receptor cross talk	Yes	No	No

Ref: [15]

Palonosetron does not inhibit or induce cytochrome P450 isoenzymes at clinically relative concentrations and has a low potential for drug interactions. Its route of excretion is equally contributed by renal and hepatic function [9, 11]. Total body clearance of palonosetron is not significantly affected by gender, age, hepatic impairment, renal impairment, or concomitant medications [21]. Palonosetron is physically and chemically stable in common infusion solutions in PVC bags and is stable when administered with dexamethasone in syringes and PVC bags.

4.2 Safety

Palonosetron exhibits the same class-related adverse affects as the first-generation 5-HT$_3$ RAs. In a meta-analysis of safety signals [22], there was no statistical difference between palonosetron and other agents in rates of constipation, headache, and diarrhea, the most common treatment-emergent adverse events. Dizziness was statistically less common in patients receiving palonosetron, OR 2.15, 95 % CI 1.05–4.41, $p=0.04$.

Prolongation of the QTc interval has been recognized as a toxicity of some of the first-generation antagonists. Palonosetron has been carefully evaluated for cardiac effects in cancer patients. Several groups have reported no significant difference in a variety of electrocardiographic parameters, including the QTc interval [23–25]. Three RCTs of palonosetron vs. other 5-HT$_3$ RAs included in the meta-analysis demonstrated minimal and significantly less mean QTc interval prolongation for palonosetron, $p=0.002$ [22].

4.3 Clinical Development of Palonosetron

A phase 2 dose-ranging study was performed with weight-based single IV dosing [26]. Complete response rates in the 40–50 % range were observed with doses ranging from 3 to 90 mcg/kg. Pharmacokinetic studies revealed a prolonged plasma half-life of approximately 40 h. Based on this trial, dose selection for the phase 3 trials was selected at fixed doses of 0.25 mg (approximately 3 mcg/kg) and 0.75 mg (approximately 10 mcg/kg).

Palonosetron was compared to the first-generation 5-HT$_3$ RAs in two multicentered multinational randomized double-blind phase 3 studies with identical study designs utilizing moderately emetogenic chemotherapy (MEC) including anthracyclines and cyclophosphamide [27, 28]. Patients received a single IV dose of palonosetron, either 0.25 mg or 0.75 mg intravenously, or ondansetron 32 mg IV as the active comparator in study 1 or dolasetron 100 mg IV in study 2. The primary endpoint for each of these trials was complete response (CR), defined as no emesis and no use of rescue medication, during the acute phase lasting 0–24 h from chemotherapy. Secondary endpoints included complete response and complete control (CC), defined as no emesis, no use of rescue medications, and no significant nausea in the delayed phase, from 24 to

120 h after chemotherapy. In the MEC-1 trial about half of the patients had breast cancer and two-thirds received cyclophosphamide with half also receiving anthracyclines [27]. The acute phase CR rate was 81 % for palonosetron 0.25 mg compared to 69 % for ondansetron, and the delayed CR rate was 75 % for palonosetron vs. 55 % for ondansetron both endpoints statistically significant. The overall phase CR rates for palonosetron were 69 % vs. 50 %, with all endpoints statistically significant. Complete control was improved in the delayed and overall phases, and number of emetic episodes was significantly reduced with superiority for palonosetron as well. Treatment-related adverse events were similar across arms: approximately 5 % of patients in both palonosetron and ondansetron arms experienced headaches, 1.6–3.2 % had constipation, and a few patients in each arm experienced dizziness.

The MEC-2 trial had an identical design except the active comparator was dolasetron [28]. Additional prophylactic corticosteroids were permitted in this study, but only 5.4 % of patients received such in a balanced fashion. In MEC-2, two-thirds of patients had breast cancer and half received AC. Complete response was 63.0 % vs. 52.9 % in the acute phase, 54.0 % vs. 38.7 % in the delayed phase, both statistically significant and also significant for the overall phase, 46.0 % vs. 34.0 % for palonosetron 0.25 mg vs. dolasetron, respectively. Significantly improved CC rate in the delayed phase and overall 5-day period study were also observed. Suppression of all emesis was statistically significant superior at all time points for palonosetron vs. dolasetron. Toxicity was similar across arms, but in MEC-2 more headache, 14.6–16.5 %, and constipation, 6.2–9.2 %, were reported. A pooled analysis of the two MEC studies [29] revealed 72 % complete response rate for palonosetron 0.25 mg compared to 60.6 % for the first-generation comparator, 64.0 % vs. 46.8 % in delayed phase and 57.7 % vs. 42.0 % overall, all statistically significant at $p < 0.025$.

The highly emetogenic (HEC) trial compared palonosetron at both doses of 0.25 mg and 0.75 mg to ondansetron 32 mg IV as the active comparator [30]. Two-thirds of patients in this study received corticosteroids in addition to the 5-HT$_3$ RA. The majority of patients received cisplatin chemotherapy at ≥ 60 mg/m^2. Overall, neither dose of palonosetron achieved a statistically significantly higher delayed complete response rate than ondansetron, but numerically a slight advantage was seen for both doses. For patients receiving concomitant dexamethasone on day 1, both delayed and acute CR rates were significantly better for palonosetron 0.25 mg. Delayed and overall emesis rates were also significantly better for palonosetron.

A study conducted by Saito et al. in Japan [31] compared palonosetron at the 0.75 mg dose plus dexamethasone to granisetron plus dexamethasone with co-primary endpoints of noninferiority of CR rates during the acute phase and superiority during the delayed phase. Patients received anthracycline and cyclophosphamide (43 % of participants) or cisplatin-based regimens (57 %). The large majority of patients were chemotherapy naïve. In this study of 1,114 patients, acute CR rates were nearly identical, 75.3 % for palonosetron and 73.3 % for granisetron, statistically noninferior, while delayed CR rate was 56.8 % for palonosetron compared to 44.5 % for granisetron ($p < 0.0001$). Overall CR rates were superior as well 51.5 % vs. 40.4 % for palonosetron vs. granisetron, respectively ($p = 0.0001$). Prespecified AC and cisplatin subsets showed similar, significant improvement with palonosetron similar to the overall study population. Nausea and emesis control was also better during the delayed phase in the palonosetron arm. Adverse events were comparable to the US/EU registrational trials in MEC. Repeat cycle analysis for the HEC trial demonstrated control maintained through four observed cycles. Similar results were reported in follow-up trials of HEC [32] and MEC [33].

Meta-analyses have been conducted for all of the randomized trials to compare the 0.75 mg and 0.25 mg doses. Therapeutic efficacy is statistically and clinically equivalent [74]. Therefore, the lowest fully effective dose, 0.25 mg IV, which is also the approved dose in US/EU, is preferred [34]. Based on the results of the phase 3 trials, palonosetron was approved by various regulatory agencies for use as prophylaxis for CINV. The current US FDA label states it palonosetron is indicated for the prevention of acute and delayed nausea and vomiting associated with initial and repeat course of both MEC and HEC in adults [21].

A patient level systematic review aggregated the data from four phase 3 studies of palonosetron $\pm$ dexamethasone compared to first-generation 5-HT$_3$ RAs for patients receiving HEC or MEC [75]. Palonosetron showed higher CR rates in pooled dose analysis during the delayed phase ($P<0.0001$) an overall phase, $p=0.0001$ but not the acute phase $p=0.091$ with similar results seen for complete control (Fig. 4.2). Results for control of emesis and nausea by severity are shown in Fig. 4.3.

4.4   Alternative Formulations

An oral form of palonosetron has also been developed and compared in a prospective, randomized dose finding study to the IV formulation. Oral palonosetron was tested at doses ranging from 0.25 to 0.75 mg, while the comparative was 0.25 mg IV following MEC [35]. The study also randomized patients to receive concurrent dexamethasone or not. While the CR rates in all arms were similar numerically, the 0.5 mg PO dose was best and most comparable to the IV dosing in the delayed and overall phases. The 0.5 mg PO dose also yielded the best results for controlling emesis and nausea. The frequency and severity of all adverse events were similar for the oral doses and the IV dose. This study established comparability between oral palonosetron at 0.50 mg and the IV formulation at 0.25 mg IV. In addition, there was no evidence for a dose response for the oral formulation within the ranges tested, paralleling the results with the IV formulation.

A subsequent randomized trial in cisplatin-based HEC compared the 0.5 mg PO dose with 0.25 mg IV [36]. Noninferiority of oral palonosetron was demonstrated in the acute phase with CR rates of 89 % for oral and 86 % for IV. Treatment-related adverse events were numerically less for the oral formulation. Together, these trials have established oral palonosetron 0.5 mg PO as therapeutically equivalent to the IV formulation of the drug.

Additionally, subcutaneous palonosetron has been tested vs. IV in a small group of patients receiving cisplatin in a cross-over design [37]. The PK parameters were

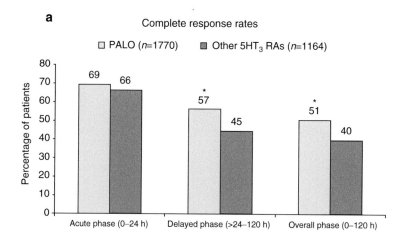

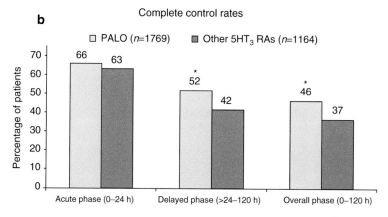

Fig. 4.2 (**a**) Comparison of palonosetron to other 5-HT$_3$ RAs, complete response = no emetic episodes and no usage of rescue medication, $p < 0.0001$ palonosetron vs. other 5-HT$_3$ RAs. (**b**) Complete control = no emetic episodes, no usage of rescue medication, and no more than mild nausea, $p < 0.0001$ palonosetron vs. other 5-HT$_3$ RAs [75]

similar for the subcutaneous formulation for area under the curve although Cmax was lower. This method of administration might be useful in certain circumstances.

4.5 Multiple-Day Chemotherapy

The best way to utilize palonosetron in the setting of multiple-day chemotherapy has been the subject of some controversy. NCCN guidelines recommend a single dose of palonosetron at the beginning of a 3-day chemotherapy regimen as an alternative to multiple daily doses of other first-generation 5-HT$_3$ receptor antagonists

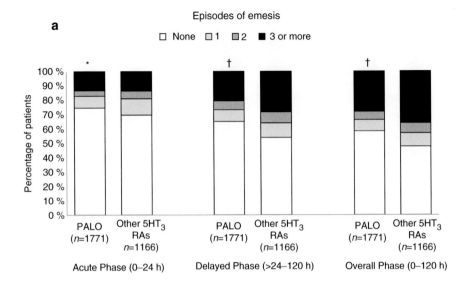

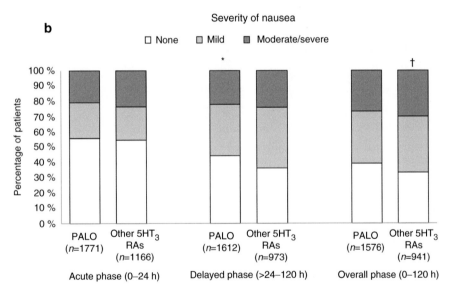

Fig. 4.3 (**a**) Episodes of emesis in the acute, delayed, and overall postchemotherapy phases. *PALO* palonesetron, *other 5-HT₃ RAs*, (ondansetron, dolasetron, and granisetron), *p=0.0066; palonosetron vs. *other 5-HT₃ RAs*; +p <0.0001 palonosetron vs. other 5-HT₃ RAs. (**b**) Severity of nausea in the acute, delayed and overall postchemotherapy phases. *PALO* palonesetron, *other 5-HT3 RAs* (ondansetron, dolasetron, and granisetron); *p=0.0002 palonosetron vs. *other 5-HT₃ RAs*; +p =0.0112 palonosetron vs. *other 5-HT₃ RAs*. [75]

[38]. The database supporting any given alternative schedule for palonosetron is scant, as few randomized trials have been performed [39]. A small pilot trial on palonosetron on days 1, 3, and 5 plus dexamethasone in men receiving 5-day cisplatin-based chemotherapy showed good control during the period of chemotherapy and for 3 days subsequently [40]. A study of palonosetron on day 1 of multiple dosing chemotherapy for hematologic malignancies showed better control compared to a retrospective review of patients treated with ondansetron [41]. Additionally in patients who experienced delayed CINV after multiple-day chemotherapy, there was better response to an additional dose of palonosetron.

In patients receiving high-dose chemotherapy, including both myeloablative and nonmyeloablative regimens over a multiple-day cycle, palonosetron and dexamethasone on day 1 was followed by dexamethasone daily and palonosetron every other day [42]. Overall complete control rates with this regimen were encouraging at 81 % and superior to case-matched controls receiving ondansetron and dexamethasone at 50 %. The use of palonosetron and longer duration of high-dose chemotherapy were independent predictors for an increased likelihood of emesis role.

Other studies [43–46] have also examined palonosetron in the setting of multiday high-dose chemotherapy programs as conditioning prior to stem cell transplant and have shown promising results in pilot trials. The best dose and schedule to utilize palonosetron in this setting remains to be determined. A triple-drug combination of aprepitant, palonosetron, and dexamethasone was more effective than palonosetron plus dexamethasone or ondansetron plus dexamethasone as prophylaxis prior to BEAM chemotherapy in non-Hodgkin's and Hodgkin's disease patients undergoing transplant [47].

4.6 Triplet CINV Prophylaxis Regimens including Palonosetron

The addition of an NK1 antagonist to a 5-HT$_3$ RA improves control of delayed CINV [48]. Aprepitant in oral or IV form (fosaprepitant) is an approved NK1 antagonist for this purpose. Aprepitant has been tested along with palonosetron and dexamethasone in a number of trials. A multicenter, single-arm phase II study enrolled patients with MEC including AC demonstrated a 78 % overall CR rate [49] for palonosetron and dexamethasone on day 1 with oral aprepitant on days 1–3. A randomized double-blind multicenter pilot trial randomized patients to palonosetron and aprepitant on day 1 only, palonosetron plus aprepitant on days 1–3, or palonosetron with placebo on days 1–3, each arm receiving dexamethasone on days 1–3 [50]. The arm without aprepitant was terminated for lack of efficacy with an approximate 50 % CR rate. Similar results were seen in the other two arms with aprepitant added on day 1 or for 3 days. A single-day triplet regimen with a dose of aprepitant equivalent to the full 3-day dose showed 76 % CR rate in acute phase and 66 % in delayed phase with no increased toxicity [51].

The triple-drug regimen was utilized in a homogenous population of lung cancer patients receiving HEC with cisplatin [52]. Complete response rates were evaluated for up to six cycles. Palonosetron, aprepitant, and dexamethasone were effective in this population with CR rates ranging from 74 % in cycle 1 to 82 % in the sixth cycle. Emesis was prevented in 90 % of patients across all cycles demonstrating the value of adding the NK1 antagonist to the combination of palonosetron and dexamethasone.

A Japanese trial compared palonosetron 0.75 mg, aprepitant, and dexamethasone to granisetron, aprepitant, and dexamethasone in 827 patients with cisplatin-based HEC [53]. CR rates were identical during the acute phase and statistically significantly higher for the delayed phase: 67 % vs. 59 % for palonosetron vs. granisetron, respectively. The overall CR rate, the primary endpoint for this trial, demonstrated superiority for palonosetron, 66 % vs. 59 %, $p = 0.01$. The three-drug regimen with aprepitant has also been studied in gynecologic patients receiving HEC, a group that is traditionally difficult to control, with an overall CR rate of 54 % [54]. Palonosetron, aprepitant, and dexamethasone have been evaluated in patients receiving multiple-day chemotherapy in small trials with efficacy established over 3- or 5-day cisplatin regimens with CR rates of 58–90 % [55, 56]. The combination of a 5-HT$_3$ RA and an NK1 RA appears to be cost-effective for the prevention of CINV [57].

Other agents other than NK1 RAs can be substituted to aid protection against delayed nausea and vomiting. Palonosetron has also been studied in combination with olanzapine, an atypical antipsychotic agent with activity against CINV [58]. A randomized trial comparing palonosetron plus dexamethasone plus aprepitant to palonosetron plus dexamethasone plus olanzapine showed no significant difference in CR rates but less nausea in the olanzapine arm in the delayed and overall phases [59]. Toxicity was similar between olanzapine and aprepitant. Olanzapine is therefore an acceptable alternative to an NK1 antagonist for patient in whom a triplet regimen is indicated as noted in the NCCN guidelines.

4.7 Role of Dexamethasone in Delayed Phase after Palonosetron

Given the activity of palonosetron and aprepitant in the delayed phase, studies have evaluated the incremental benefit of dexamethasone given beyond day 1. Dexamethasone is associated with significant side effects when given in antiemetic doses for prolonged periods, including insomnia, gastrointestinal distress, exacerbation of diabetes mellitus, and weight gain. Given the benefit of aprepitant in the delayed phase of CINV, a randomized comparison of dexamethasone vs. aprepitant beyond day 1 in patients receiving AC was conducted [60]. Complete response rates were similar during the acute phase and were identical at 79.5 % during the delayed phase. Significantly less insomnia, heartburn, and improved functional living scores were noted for the aprepitant arm. As such, palonosetron with IV aprepitant and dexamethasone on day 1 or oral aprepitant on days 1–3 appears a reasonable alternative to continuing dexamethasone in patients receiving AC.

Several trials have evaluated palonosetron plus dexamethasone on day 1 vs. continuing dexamethasone on days 2 and 3 in patients receiving AC and/or other MEC regimens. Three noninferiority trials demonstrated no significant difference achieved in each of these studies [61–63]. Therefore, when using palonosetron and dexamethasone as a doublet in non-AC MEC, it appears that the regimen can be limited to a simplified day 1 prophylactic program without sacrificing efficacy but reducing toxicity.

4.8   Cost-Effectiveness of Palonosetron

The cost of cancer care has skyrocketed over the past decade and appears unsustainable [64]. Each new improvement in cancer care, whether therapeutic or supportive in nature, is appropriately subject to scrutiny regarding the cost-effectiveness of the intervention. Standards are slowly emerging to establish value parameters in healthcare with thresholds set for improvement per unit cost.

To this end, the cost of prophylaxis against CINV has been subjected to cost-effectiveness analyses. It is clear that non-prevented CINV events are associated with significant cost to individual patients, families, and the healthcare system as a whole. One retrospective cohort study of over 19,000 adult patients receiving HEC or MEC with CINV prophylaxis examined the cost of uncontrolled CINV [65]. In this cohort 13.8 % of patients had a CINV-associated healthcare visit. Resource utilization included inpatient admissions, unscheduled outpatient visits, and emergency room visits. The mean per-patient CINV-associated cost across all patients treated was $731.00. The mean cost of a CINV event to an individual patient was $5,299.00. Another US study showed a healthcare resource cost in a hospital outpatient setting of $1,855.00 [66]. Despite differences in methodology and cost figures presented by these analyses, there can be no doubt that CINV events are associated with more cost to the healthcare system.

Therefore, strategies that control CINV better are likely to reduce healthcare costs for downstream CINV events. A cost-utility assessment using quality-adjusted life-years (QALY) as the value parameter compared palonosetron to ondansetron ± aprepitant in a Monte Carlo simulation model [67]. Incremental cost-effectiveness for the palonosetron regimens was $115,490/QALY for the two-drug regimen, $199,375/QALY for the palonosetron plus aprepitant plus dexamethasone regimen, and $200,525/QALY for the three-drug strategy vs. the ondansetron-based two-drug regimen. These QALYs are in the range of acceptability. Whether QALY is the right metric to use for a supportive care drug that is used broadly is subject to debate; however, even in this context these costs for QALYs are similar to newer biological agents designed for therapeutic intent.

A retrospective analysis of the OptumInsight claims database from years 2005 to 2011, comprised largely of commercially insured members, revealed delayed CINV of 15.6 % across all cycles, utilizing all 5-HT3 receptor antagonists [68]. The lowest rates were demonstrated in patients receiving palonosetron. Over six cycles of chemotherapy per 1,000 patients, ondansetron costs an additional $126,775 and granisetron an additional $169,838 compared to using palonosetron from cycle 1. In a hospital outpatient setting, patients receiving palonosetron had a 14 % decreased rate of CINV per chemotherapy cycle [69].

A systemic review of the literature surrounding cost analyses of CINV in relation to 5-HT$_3$ receptor antagonist utilized was published in 2014 [70]. Thirty-two studies were analyzed including randomized controlled trials. Fourteen reported cost data and 25 studies utilization data. Palonosetron was associated with higher acquisition and treatment costs in the first-generation 5-HT$_3$ RAs. However, healthcare utilization for CINV was reduced in patients receiving palonosetron due to the less need for rescue medication and downstream services such as outpatient visits and emergency room visits. Therefore, the overall costs associated with using palonosetron as the 5-HT$_3$ receptor antagonist of choice appear to be lower than other agents due to reduced service utilization for CINV.

4.9 Pediatric Use

Palonosetron has not been extensively studied in the pediatric population. Retrospective comparison of palonosetron to first-generation 5-HT$_3$ RAs in children showed a significant reduction in emesis on the first 3 days and nausea in the first 4 days in the palonosetron group [71]. A retrospective analysis of children undergoing BMT revealed 43 patients who received palonosetron in a dose of 5 mcg/kg. CINV was controlled in 68 %. A second dose of palonosetron was required on day 5 of the underlying regimen in 17 % of patients [72]. A prospective observational trial examined palonosetron at 5 mcg/kg in children with ALL receiving high-dose methotrexate 5 g/m^2. CR was achieved in 84 % in the acute phase and 60 % overall with 90 % free of emesis [73]. Palonosetron is approved in the USA for pediatric use for the prevention of CINV at a dose of 20 mcg/kg [21].

4.10 Meta-Analysis

Several systematic reviews in meta-analysis have been conducted comparing the efficacy and toxicity of the 5-HT$_3$ RAs to one another. Likun reviewed eight RCTs involving 3,592 patients published between 2003 and 2010 [74]. Most trials were noninferiority studies comparing first-generation agents to palonosetron alone. Overall, palonosetron showed superiority for complete response rate with an odds ratio of 0.64 (95 % CI, 0.56–0.74, $p < 0.00001$). In two studies with HEC comparing palonosetron and dexamethasone to first-generation 5-HT$_3$ RAs plus dexamethasone, there was a trend in favor of palonosetron for acute CINV and statistical benefit for palonosetron in delayed and overall phase. For MEC, palonosetron was superior to prevent acute CINV with an OR of 0.70 (95 % CI, 0.54–0.91, $p=0.008$), delayed CINV, and nausea.

The most recent meta-analysis, published in 2014 by Popovic et.al., identified 16 RCTs with over 6,000 patients randomized to palonesetron or other 5-HT$_3$ RAs [22]. Multiple endpoints were analyzed including complete response, complete control, no emesis, no nausea, and no use of rescue medications. Of note, only one of the trials included aprepitant; so this analysis serves as a direct comparison of 5-HT$_3$ RAs to palonosetron alone or as doublet therapy with corticosteroids. Acute, delayed, and overall phases were analyzed separately.

Palonosetron showed statistically significant superiority in the overall phase of CINV for all five endpoints, with odds ratios ranging from 1.51 to 1.54 for each of the endpoints. In subgroup analysis, palonosetron was superior for CR whether or not patients received concomitant corticosteroids. Evaluation by level of emetogenicity demonstrated palonosetron superiority in both HEC and MEC for complete response,

Table 4.2 Absolute risk differences between palonosetron and other 5-hydroxytryptamine 3 receptor antagonist intervention arms for all included chemotherapy-induced nausea and vomiting endpoints [22]

Endpoint	Absolute risk Difference (% @ 95 % CI)	Test for overall effect	Satisfies MASCC/ESMO antiemetic guideline requirement
CR, acute phase	6 (3–8)	$p=0.0001$	No
CR, delayed phase	12 (9–15)	$p<0.00001$	Yes
Cr, overall phase	10 (7–14)	$p<0.00001$	Approaching requirement
CC, acute phase	6 (2–9)	$p=0.0008$	No
CC, delayed phase	11 (8–15)	$p<0.00001$	Yes
CC, overall phase	11 (7–14)	$p<0.00001$	Yes
No emesis, acute phase	5 (2–8)	$p=0.02$	No
No emesis, delayed phase	10 (7–14)	$p<0.0001$	Approaching requirement
No emesis, overall phase	10 (7–14)	$p>0.00001$	Approaching requirement
No nausea, acute phase	4 (0–9)	$p=0.03$	No
No nausea, delayed phase	8 (3–12)	$p=0.0008$	Approaching requirement
No nausea, overall phase	9 (4–13)	$p=0.0003$	Approaching requirement
No rescue medications, acute phase	5 (−5 to 16)	$p=0.32$	No
No rescue medications, delayed phase	6 (−1 to 13)	$p=0.12$	No
No rescue medications, overall phase	8 (2–14)	$p=0.01$	Approaching requirement

MASCC Multinational Association of Supportive Care in Cancer, *ESMO* European Society of Medical Oncology, *CR* complete response, *CC* complete control complete control, and no emesis endpoints. Palonosetron was also statistically superior in both the acute and delayed phases for CR, CC, no emesis, and no nausea.

MASCC/ESMO guidelines suggest an absolute risk difference of 10 % between antiemetic regimens as a level constituting a clinically relevant result that could prompt guideline revision [76, 77]. Table 4.2 shows the results of the meta-analysis by each of the endpoints for overall, acute, and delayed phases. Of the 15 prespecified endpoints, 3 meet the MASCC/ESMO criteria and 6 approach it. Taken together, the meta-analysis demonstrates that the weight of the evidence from randomized clinical trials conducted over the past decade strongly favors palonosetron as more efficacious in preventing CINV compared to first-generation 5-HT$_3$ RAs.

This study also provided a comprehensive evaluation of safety of the various 5-HT$_3$ RAs. Palonosetron was statistically similar to the other agents with regard to constipation, headache, and diarrhea and safer with regard to dizziness. Evaluation of the three RCTs reporting mean QTc interval change revealed palonosetron was significantly safer than the comparator 5-HT$_3$ RAs with less overall change in QTc interval after drug administration.

4.11 Palonosetron in Antiemetic Guidelines

Multiple guidelines have been created to collate evidence-based recommendations to cancer treatment, including CINV prophylaxis. While the methodology and the frequency of updating vary somewhat, the various organizations use tiered evidence bases +/− expert opinion to generate the recommendations. Recommendations for HEC and MEC from each of these guideline groups are shown in Figs. 4.4 and 4.5. All guidelines recommend palonosetron as the 5-HT$_3$ RA of choice in MEC [38, 77, 78]. In HEC, all guidelines recommend a three drug combination, consisting of a 5-HT$_3$ RA, dexamethasone and an NK1 antagonist (or, in NCCN, olanzapine). Conforming to guideline recommendations improves CINV control; unfortunately adherence remains suboptimal [79, 80]. New strategies to promote guideline usage through educational efforts, and improved awareness of patient experience following chemotherapy by clinicians, possibly using electronic tools, could help this situation [81].

4.12 Netupitant and Palonosetron (NEPA) Fixed Combination

Netupitant is a highly selective NK1 RA which exhibits a high degree of receptor occupancy [81]. In vitro studies have shown a synergistic effect in preventing NK1 response to substance P [20] and an additive effect on NK1 receptor internalization [15]. The plasma half-life of netupitant is approximately 96 h, suggesting

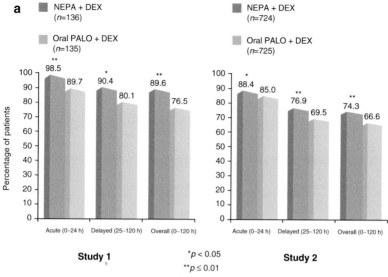

Cycle 1 complete response (no emesis, no rescue medication) rates
NEPA vs. oral palonosetron (studies 1 & 2)

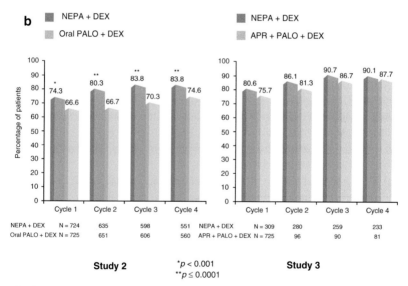

Overall (0–120 h) complete response (no emesis, no rescue
medication rates over multiple chemotherapy cycles:
NEPA vs. oral palonosetron (study 2) & NEPA vs. aprepitant regimen (study 3)

Fig. 4.4 (**a**) Complete response to NEPA vs. oral palonosetron in cycle 1. *Study 1* = dosing-finding study. *Study 2* = MEC. (**b**) Complete response to NEPA vs. other comparators across multiple cycles. *Study 2* = MEC. *Study 3* = NEPA + dexamethasone vs. palonosetron + aprepitant + dexamethasone [81]

MEC: Guideline Recommendations

	Acute CINV	Delayed CINV (d 2-3)
NCCN	Palo + Dex +/- NK1* Or Olanzapine + Palo + Dex	5 HT3 (if Palo not used d1) or Dex or APR* +/- Dex or Olanzapine#
ASCO	Palo + Dex	Dex
MASCC	Palo + Dex	Dex

HEC: Guideline Recommendations

	Acute CINV	Delayed CINV (d 2-3)	Delayed CINV (d 4)
NCCN	5HT3 + Dex + NK1 Or NEPA + Dex Or Olanzapine + Palo + Dex	Dex + APR* Or Olanzapine#	Dex
ASCO	5HT3 + Dex + APR Or NEPA + Dex	Dex + APR*	Dex
MASCC	5HT3 + Dex + APR	Dex + APR*	

Palo: Palonosetron APR: Aprepitant
NK1: Aprepitant, fosaprepitant or rolapitant, or NEPA (no additional palo)
*If fosaprepitant used, day 1 only
#If olanzapine used on day 1

NK1: Aprepitant, fosaprepitant or rolapitant or NEPA (no additional 5HT3)
APR: Aprepitant
*If fosaprepitant or NEPA used, Dex only on days 2-4
#If olanzapine used on day 1

Fig. 4.5 Guideline recommendations

that there could be a clinical benefit in the delayed phase of CINV when coadministered with palonosetron. Netupitant is a substrate and moderate inhibitor of CYP3A4. Drugs that are substrates of CYP3A4, such as dexamethasone, should be administered in reduced doses when given with netupitant. Unlike aprepitant, netupitant does not have clinically relevant interactions with oral contraceptives, and no relevant PK interactions are seen when netupitant is co-administered with palonosetron [82].

NEPA has a similar adverse event profile to oral palonosetron given with aprepitant with headache and constipation the most frequently observed toxicities. A comprehensive review of NEPA safety revealed similar treatment-emergent adverse events for NEPA, oral palonosetron alone, or palonosetron and aprepitant combination [83]. No significant effect on QTc interval or impact on other cardiac endpoints was observed across various studies.

NEPA has been evaluated in three trials conducted across a range of emetogenicity in chemotherapy-naïve patients. A phase 2 dose-ranging study compared three different doses of netupitant combined with oral palonosetron to oral palonosetron alone in 694 patients receiving cisplatin-based chemotherapy [84]. The 300 mg dose of netupitant was selected for further evaluation based on numerical superiority in CR rate. Additionally, 300 mg of netupitant was the minimal dose demonstrating NK1 receptor occupancy of >90 % in the brain striatum, the accepted value for efficacy, in a previously performed pharmacodynamic PET study [85]. Overall, NEPA was significantly superior to oral palonosetron for CR in acute, delayed, and overall phases (Fig. 4.4a, Study 1).

A phase 3, multinational double-blind placebo-controlled trial evaluated oral NEPA + dexamethasone compared to oral palonosetron + dexamethasone in 1,455 patients receiving AC-based chemotherapy [86]. Significant improvement in CR rate during the delayed phase of cycle 1, the primary endpoint of the trial, was seen with 77 % of the NEPA group compared to 69 % of the palonosetron group, $p = 0.001$. Additionally, overall phase CR rate was 74 % vs. 67 %, $p = 0.001$, and acute phase CR rate was 88 % vs. 85 %, $p = 0.047$ for NEPA vs. palonosetron, respectively (Fig. 4.4a, Study 2). In other endpoints including delayed and overall phases, no emesis, no significant nausea, and complete protection statistically significant higher rates were also achieved.

A multiple cycle trial in HEC and MEC was conducted primarily to assess cumulative safety [87]. This study included an arm of oral palonosetron and aprepitant compared to NEPA, with both arms receiving dexamethasone according to guidelines. The overall phase CR rate in cycle 1 was 81 % for NEPA and 76 % for palonosetron and aprepitant. No formal statistical comparison was performed. Antiemetic efficacy was maintained well over multiple cycles of therapy, as was also seen in an analysis of the multiple cycle extension study of NEPA during MEC [88] (Fig. 4.4b). NEPA was approved by the US FDA in 2014 for the prevention of acute and delayed nausea and vomiting associated with initial and repeat course of chemotherapy including, but not limited to, highly emetogenic chemotherapy [89]. NEPA is included in NCCN and ASCO guidelines as a prophylactic choice for HEC and MEC.

While NEPA has not yet been subjected to formal cost-effectiveness analyses, the superiority of NEPA over a two-drug regimen on a clinical basis supports the value. The appropriate formal comparison would be NEPA plus dexamethasone to palonosetron with aprepitant and dexamethasone. The fact that NEPA is a fixed combination suggests a potential economic benefit as adherence to fixed dose combinations in general is associated with improved adherence and lower overall treatment cost [57].

4.13 Conclusion

Palonosetron differs chemically, pharmacologically, and, most importantly, clinically from the first-generation 5-HT_3 RAs. It confers significant additional protection against delayed nausea and vomiting and in the overall phase of CINV. Multiple prospective randomized trials have demonstrated the benefit of palonosetron over first-generation agents in patients receiving MEC, AC, and HEC regimens. Adding an NK1 antagonist appears to increase the response rate to palonosetron and dexamethasone. Palonosetron is equally effective in IV and oral formulations and is now available in a fixed combination with the NK1 RA netupitant which offers increased convenience and the potential for better adherence.

References

1. Geling O, Eichler HG (2005) Should 5-hydroxytryptamine-3 receptor antagonists be administered beyond 24 hours after chemotherapy to prevent delayed emesis? Systematic re-evaluation of clinical evidence and drug cost implications. J Clin Oncol Off J Am Soc Clin Oncol 23(6):1289–1294

2. Hickok JT, Roscoe JA, Morrow GR et al (2005) 5-Hydroxytryptamine-receptor antagonists versus prochlorperazine for control of delayed nausea caused by doxorubicin: a URCC CCOP randomised controlled trial. Lancet Oncol 6(10):765–772
3. Gralla RJ, Navari RM, Hesketh PJ et al (1998) Single-dose oral granisetron has equivalent antiemetic efficacy to intravenous ondansetron for highly emetogenic cisplatin-based chemotherapy. J Clin Oncol Off J Am Soc Clin Oncol 16(4):1568–1573
4. Perez EA, Hesketh P, Sandbach J et al (1998) Comparison of single-dose oral granisetron versus intravenous ondansetron in the prevention of nausea and vomiting induced by moderately emetogenic chemotherapy: a multicenter, double-blind, randomized parallel study. J Clin Oncol Off J Am Soc Clin Oncol 16(2):754–760
5. Clark RD, Miller AB, Berger J et al (1993) 2-(Quinuclidin-3-yl)pyrido[4,3-b]indol-1-ones and isoquinolin-1-ones. Potent conformationally restricted 5-HT3 receptor antagonists. J Med Chem 36(18):2645–2657
6. Yan D, Schulte MK, Bloom KE, White MM (1999) Structural features of the ligand-binding domain of the serotonin 5HT3 receptor. J Biol Chem 274(9):5537–5541
7. Eglen RM, Lee CH, Smith WL et al (1995) Pharmacological characterization of RS 25259-197, a novel and selective 5-HT3 receptor antagonist, in vivo. Br J Pharmacol 114(4):860–866
8. Wong EH, Clark R, Leung E et al (1995) The interaction of RS 25259-197, a potent and selective antagonist, with 5-HT3 receptors, in vitro. Br J Pharmacol 114(4):851–859
9. Stoltz R, Cyong JC, Shah A, Parisi S (2004) Pharmacokinetic and safety evaluation of palonosetron, a 5-hydroxytryptamine-3 receptor antagonist, in U.S. and Japanese healthy subjects. J Clin Pharmacol 44(5):520–531
10. Constenla M (2004) 5-HT3 receptor antagonists for prevention of late acute-onset emesis. Ann Pharmacother 38(10):1683–1691
11. Stoltz R, Parisi S, Shah A, Macciocchi A (2004) Pharmacokinetics, metabolism and excretion of intravenous [14C]-palonosetron in healthy human volunteers. Biopharm Drug Dispos 25(8):329–337
12. Rojas C, Stathis M, Thomas AG et al (2008) Palonosetron exhibits unique molecular interactions with the 5-HT3 receptor. Anesth Analg 107(2):469–478
13. Rojas C, Thomas AG, Alt J et al (2010) Palonosetron triggers 5-HT(3) receptor internalization and causes prolonged inhibition of receptor function. Eur J Pharmacol 626(2–3):193–199
14. Rojas C, Slusher BS (2012) Pharmacological mechanisms of 5-HT(3) and tachykinin NK(1) receptor antagonism to prevent chemotherapy-induced nausea and vomiting. Eur J Pharmacol 684(1–3):1–7
15. Rojas C, Raje M, Tsukamoto T, Slusher BS (2014) Molecular mechanisms of 5-HT(3) and NK(1) receptor antagonists in prevention of emesis. Eur J Pharmacol 722:26–37
16. Hothersall JD, Moffat C, Connolly CN (2013) Prolonged inhibition of 5-HT(3) receptors by palonosetron results from surface receptor inhibition rather than inducing receptor internalization. Br J Pharmacol 169(6):1252–1262
17. Darmani NA, Chebolu S, Amos B, Alkam T (2011) Synergistic antiemetic interactions between serotonergic 5-HT3 and tachykininergic NK1-receptor antagonists in the least shrew (Cryptotis parva). Pharmacol Biochem Behav 99(4):573–579
18. Minami M, Endo T, Yokota H et al (2001) Effects of CP-99, 994, a tachykinin NK(1) receptor antagonist, on abdominal afferent vagal activity in ferrets: evidence for involvement of NK(1) and 5-HT(3) receptors. Eur J Pharmacol 428(2):215–220
19. Hu WP, You XH, Guan BC, Ru LQ, Chen JG, Li ZW (2004) Substance P potentiates 5-HT3 receptor-mediated current in rat trigeminal ganglion neurons. Neurosci Lett 365(2):147–152
20. Stathis M, Pietra C, Rojas C, Slusher BS (2012) Inhibition of substance P-mediated responses in NG108-15 cells by netupitant and palonosetron exhibit synergistic effects. Eur J Pharmacol 689(1–3):25–30
21. Aloxi prescribing information (2015) Accessed 12.7.15 www.Aloxi.com/docs/pdf/pi.pdf
22. Popovic M, Warr DG, Deangelis C et al (2014) Efficacy and safety of palonosetron for the prophylaxis of chemotherapy-induced nausea and vomiting (CINV): a systematic review and

meta-analysis of randomized controlled trials. Support Care Cancer Off J Multinatl Assoc Support Care Cancer 22(6):1685–1697

23. Yavas C, Dogan U, Yavas G, Araz M, Ata OY (2012) Acute effect of palonosetron on electro-cardiographic parameters in cancer patients: a prospective study. Support Care Cancer Off J Multinatl Assoc Support Care Cancer 20(10):2343–2347

24. Gonullu G, Demircan S, Demirag MK, Erdem D, Yucel I (2012) Electrocardiographic findings of palonosetron in cancer patients. Support Care Cancer Off J Multinatl Assoc Support Care Cancer 20(7):1435–1439

25. Dogan U, Yavas G, Tekinalp M, Yavas C, Ata OY, Ozdemir K (2012) Evaluation of the acute effect of palonosetron on transmural dispersion of myocardial repolarization. Eur Rev Med Pharmacol Sci 16(4):462–468

26. Eisenberg P, MacKintosh FR, Ritch P, Cornett PA, Macciocchi A (2004) Efficacy, safety and pharmacokinetics of palonosetron in patients receiving highly emetogenic cisplatin-based che-motherapy: a dose-ranging clinical study. Ann Oncol Off J Eur Soc Med Oncol/ESMO 15(2):330–337

27. Gralla R, Lichinitser M, Van Der Vegt S et al (2003) Palonosetron improves prevention of chemotherapy-induced nausea and vomiting following moderately emetogenic chemotherapy: results of a double-blind randomized phase III trial comparing single doses of palonosetron with ondansetron. Ann Oncol Off J Eur Soc Med Oncol/ESMO 14(10):1570–1577

28. Eisenberg P, Figueroa-Vadillo J, Zamora R et al (2003) Improved prevention of moderately emetogenic chemotherapy-induced nausea and vomiting with palonosetron, a pharmacologi-cally novel 5-HT3 receptor antagonist: results of a phase III, single-dose trial versus dolase-tron. Cancer 98(11):2473–2482

29. Celio L, Agustoni F, Testa I, Dotti K, de Braud F (2012) Palonosetron: an evidence-based choice in prevention of nausea and vomiting induced by moderately emetogenic chemother-apy. Tumori 98(3):279–286

30. Aapro MS, Grunberg SM, Manikhas GM et al (2006) A phase III, double-blind, randomized trial of palonosetron compared with ondansetron in preventing chemotherapy-induced nausea and vomiting following highly emetogenic chemotherapy. Ann Oncol Off J Eur Soc Med Oncol/ESMO 17(9):1441–1449

31. Saito M, Aogi K, Sekine I et al (2009) Palonosetron plus dexamethasone versus granisetron plus dexamethasone for prevention of nausea and vomiting during chemotherapy: a double-blind, double-dummy, randomised, comparative phase III trial. Lancet Oncol 10(2):115–124

32. Aogi K, Sakai H, Yoshizawa H et al (2012) A phase III open-label study to assess safety and efficacy of palonosetron for preventing chemotherapy-induced nausea and vomiting (CINV) in repeated cycles of emetogenic chemotherapy. Support Care Cancer Off J Multinatl Assoc Support Care Cancer 20(7):1507–1514

33. Lorusso V, Giampaglia M, Petrucelli L, Saracino V, Perrone T, Gnoni A (2012) Antiemetic efficacy of single-dose palonosetron and dexamethasone in patients receiving multiple cycles of multiple day-based chemotherapy. Support Care Cancer Off J Multinatl Assoc Support Care Cancer 20(12):3241–3246

34. Kris M, Tonato M, Bria E et al (2011) Consensus recommendations for the presentation of vomiting and nausea following high-emetic-risk chemotherapy. 19: Suppl 1:S25–32.

35. Boccia R, Grunberg S, Franco-Gonzales E, Rubenstein E, Voisin D (2013) Efficacy of oral palonosetron compared to intravenous palonosetron for the prevention of chemotherapy-induced nausea and vomiting associated with moderately emetogenic chemotherapy: a phase 3 trial. Support Care Cancer Off J Multinatl Assoc Support Care Cancer 21(5):1453–1460

36. Karthaus M, Tibor C, Lorusso V et al (2015) Efficacy and safety of oral palonesetron compared with IV palonesetron administered with dexamethasone for the prevention of chemotherapy-induced nausea and vomiting (CINV) in patients with solid tumors receiving cisplatin-based highly emetogenic chemotherapy (HEC). Support Care Cancer 23(10):2917–2923.

37. Sadaba B, del Barrio A, Campanero MA et al (2014) Randomized pharmacokinetic study comparing subcutaneous and intravenous palonosetron in cancer patients treated with plati-num based chemotherapy. PLoS One 9(2):e89747

38. NCCN Antiemesis Guidelines Version 2.2015, Accessed 12.7.15 www.nccn.org/professionals/physician_gls/pdf/antiemesis.pdf
39. Affronti ML, Bubalo J (2014) Palonosetron in the management of chemotherapy-induced nausea and vomiting in patients receiving multiple-day chemotherapy. Cancer Manag Res 6:329–337
40. Einhorn LH, Brames MJ, Dreicer R, Nichols CR, Cullen MT Jr, Bubalo J (2007) Palonosetron plus dexamethasone for prevention of chemotherapy-induced nausea and vomiting in patients receiving multiple-day cisplatin chemotherapy for germ cell cancer. Support Care Cancer Off J Multinatl Assoc Support Care Cancer 15(11):1293–1300
41. Musso M, Scalone R, Bonanno V et al (2009) Palonosetron (Aloxi) and dexamethasone for the prevention of acute and delayed nausea and vomiting in patients receiving multiple-day chemotherapy. Support Care Cancer Off J Multinatl Assoc Support Care Cancer 17(2):205–209
42. Mirabile A, Celio L, Magni M, Bonizzoni E, Gianni AM, Di Nicola M (2014) Evaluation of an every-other-day palonosetron schedule to control emesis in multiple-day high-dose chemotherapy. Future Oncol 10(16):2569–2578
43. Musso M, Scalone R, Crescimanno A et al (2010) Palonosetron and dexamethasone for prevention of nausea and vomiting in patients receiving high-dose chemotherapy with auto-SCT. Bone Marrow Transplant 45(1):123–127
44. Yeh S, Lo W, Hsieh C, Bai L et al (2014) Palonosetron and dexamethasone for the prevention of nausea and vomiting in patients receiving allogeneic hematopoietic stem cell transplantation. Support Care Cancer 22:1199–1206
45. Chou CW, Chen YK, Yu YB, Chang KH, Hwang WL, Teng CL (2014) Palonosetron versus first-generation 5-hydroxytryptamine type 3 receptor antagonists for emesis prophylaxis in patients undergoing allogeneic hematopoietic stem cell transplantation. Ann Hematol 93(7):1225–1232
46. Giralt SA, Mangan KF, Maziarz RT et al (2011) Three palonosetron regimens to prevent CINV in myeloma patients receiving multiple-day high-dose melphalan and hematopoietic stem cell transplantation. Ann Oncol Off J Eur Soc Med Oncol/ESMO 22(4):939–946
47. Pielichowski W, Barzal J, Gawronski K et al (2011) A triple-drug combination to prevent nausea and vomiting following BEAM chemotherapy before autologous hematopoietic stem cell transplantation. Transplant Proc 43(8):3107–3110
48. Navari RM (2013) Management of chemotherapy-induced nausea and vomiting: focus on newer agents and new uses for older agents. Drugs 73(3):249–262
49. Grote T, Hajdenberg J, Cartmell A, Ferguson S, Ginkel A, Charu V (2006) Combination therapy for chemotherapy-induced nausea and vomiting in patients receiving moderately emetogenic chemotherapy: palonosetron, dexamethasone, and aprepitant. J Support Oncol 4(8):403–408
50. Herrington JD, Jaskiewicz AD, Song J (2008) Randomized, placebo-controlled, pilot study evaluating aprepitant single dose plus palonosetron and dexamethasone for the prevention of acute and delayed chemotherapy-induced nausea and vomiting. Cancer 112(9):2080–2087
51. Grunberg SM, Dugan M, Muss H et al (2009) Effectiveness of a single-day three-drug regimen of dexamethasone, palonosetron, and aprepitant for the prevention of acute and delayed nausea and vomiting caused by moderately emetogenic chemotherapy. Support Care Cancer Off J Multinatl Assoc Support Care Cancer 17(5):589–594
52. Longo F, Mansueto G, Lapadula V et al (2012) Combination of aprepitant, palonosetron and dexamethasone as antiemetic prophylaxis in lung cancer patients receiving multiple cycles of cisplatin-based chemotherapy. Int J Clin Pract 66(8):753–757
53. Hashimoto H, Yamanaka T, Shimada Y et al (2013) Palonosetron (PALO) vs. granisetron (GRA) in the triplet regiment with dexamethasone (DEX) and aprepitant (APR) for preventing highly emetogenic chemotherapy (HEC) with cisplatin (CDDP): a randomized double-blind phase III trial. J Clin Oncol. 31(suppl): 9621
54. Takeshima N, Matoda M, Abe M et al (2014) Efficacy and safety of triple therapy with aprepitant, palonosetron, and dexamethasone for preventing nausea and vomiting induced by cisplatin-based chemotherapy for gynecological cancer: KCOG-G1003 phase II trial. Support Care Cancer Off J Multinatl Assoc Support Care Cancer 22(11):2891–2898

55. Gao HF, Liang Y, Zhou NN, Zhang DS, Wu HY (2013) Aprepitant plus palonosetron and dexamethasone for prevention of chemotherapy-induced nausea and vomiting in patients receiving multiple-day cisplatin chemotherapy. Intern Med J 43(1):73–76
56. Hamada S, Hinotsu S, Kawai K et al (2014) Antiemetic efficacy and safety of a combination of palonosetron, aprepitant, and dexamethasone in patients with testicular germ cell tumor receiving 5-day cisplatin-based combination chemotherapy. Support Care Cancer Off J Multinatl Assoc Support Care Cancer 22(8):2161–2166
57. Schwartzberg L (2014) Addressing the value of novel therapies in chemotherapy-induced nausea and vomiting. Expert Rev Pharmacoecon Outcomes Res 14(6):825–834
58. Ohzawa H, Miki A, Hozumi Y et al (2015) Comparison between the antiemetic effects of palonosetron and granisetron in breast cancer patients treated with anthracycline-based regimens. Oncol Lett 9(1):119–124
59. Navari R, Gray S, Kerr A (2011) Olanzapine versus aprepitant for the prevention of chemotherapy-induced nausea and vomiting: a randomized phase III trial. J Support Onc 9(5):188–195
60. Roila F, Ruggeri B, Ballatori E, Del Favero A, Tonato M (2014) Aprepitant versus dexamethasone for preventing chemotherapy-induced delayed emesis in patients with breast cancer: a randomized double-blind study. J Clin Oncol Off J Am Soc Clin Oncol 32(2):101–106
61. Aapro M, Fabi A, Nole F et al (2010) Double-blind, randomised, controlled study of the efficacy and tolerability of palonosetron plus dexamethasone for 1 day with or without dexamethasone on days 2 and 3 in the prevention of nausea and vomiting induced by moderately emetogenic chemotherapy. Ann Oncol Off J Eur Soc Med Oncol/ESMO 21(5):1083–1088
62. Komatsu Y, Okita K, Yuki S et al (2015) Open-label, randomized, comparative phase III study on effects of reducing steroid use in combination with Palonosetron. Cancer Sci 106(7):891–895
63. Celio L, Bonizzoni E, Bajetta E, Sebastiani S, Perrone T, Aapro MS (2013) Palonosetron plus single-dose dexamethasone for the prevention of nausea and vomiting in women receiving anthracycline/cyclophosphamide-containing chemotherapy: meta-analysis of individual patient data examining the effect of age on outcome in two phase III trials. Support Care Cancer Off J Multinatl Assoc Support Care Cancer 21(2):565–573
64. Kantarjian H, Rajkumar SV (2015) Why are cancer drugs so expensive in the United States, and what are the solutions? Mayo Clin Proc 90(4):500–504
65. Burke TA, Wisniewski T, Ernst FR (2011) Resource utilization and costs associated with chemotherapy-induced nausea and vomiting (CINV) following highly or moderately emetogenic chemotherapy administered in the US outpatient hospital setting. Support Care Cancer Off J Multinatl Assoc Support Care Cancer 19(1):131–140
66. Craver C, Gayle J, Balu S, Buchner D (2011) Palonosetron versus other 5-HT(3) receptor antagonists for prevention of chemotherapy-induced nausea and vomiting in patients with hematologic malignancies treated with emetogenic chemotherapy in a hospital outpatient setting in the United States. J Med Econ 14(3):341–349
67. Avritscher EB, Shih YC, Sun CC et al (2010) Cost-utility analysis of palonosetron-based therapy in preventing emesis among breast cancer patients. J Support Oncol 8(6):242–251
68. Faria C, Li X, Nagl N, McBride A (2014) Outcomes associated with 5-HT3-RA therapy selection in patients with chemotherapy-induced nausea and vomiting: a retrospective claims analysis. Am Health Drug Benefits 7(1):50–58
69. Balu S, Buchner D, Craver C, Gayle J (2011) Palonosetron versus other 5-HT(3) receptor antagonists for prevention of chemotherapy-induced nausea and vomiting in patients with cancer on chemotherapy in a hospital outpatient setting. Clin Ther 33(4):443–455
70. Broder MS, Faria C, Powers A, Sunderji J, Cherepanov D (2014) The impact of 5-HT3RA use on cost and utilization in patients with chemotherapy-induced nausea and vomiting: systematic review of the literature. Am Health Drug Benefits 7(3):171–182
71. Sepulveda-Vildosola AC, Betanzos-Cabrera Y, Lastiri GG et al (2008) Palonosetron hydrochloride is an effective and safe option to prevent chemotherapy-induced nausea and vomiting in children. Arch Med Res 39(6):601–606
72. Ripaldi M, Parasole R, De Simone G et al (2010) Palonosetron to prevent nausea and vomiting in children undergoing BMT: efficacy and safety. Bone Marrow Transplant 45(11):1663–1664

73. Nadaraja S, Mamoudou AD, Thomassen H, Wehner PS, Rosthoej S, Schroeder H (2012) Palonosetron for the prevention of nausea and vomiting in children with acute lymphoblastic leukemia treated with high dose methotrexate. Pediatr Blood Cancer 59(5):870–873
74. Likun Z, Xiang J, Yi B, Xin D, Tao ZL (2011) A systematic review and meta-analysis of intravenous palonosetron in the prevention of chemotherapy-induced nausea and vomiting in adults. Oncologist 16(2):207–216
75. Schwartzberg L, Barbour S, Morrow G et al (2014) Pooled analysis of Phase III clinical studies of palonesetron versus ondansetron, dolasetron and granisetron in the prevention of chemotherapy-induced nausea and vomiting (CINV). Support Care Cancer 22:469–477
76. Herrstedt J, Roila F, ESMO guideline working group (2009) Chemotherapy-induced nausea and vomiting: ESMO clinical recommendations for prophylaxis. Ann Oncol 20, suppl 4:156–8
77. Jordan K, Gralla R, Jahn F, Molassiotis A (2014) International antiemetic guidelines on chemotherapy induced nausea and vomiting (CINV): content and implementation in daily routine practice. Eur J Pharmacol 722:197–202
78. Hesketh P, Bohlke K, Lyman G et al (2015) Antiemetics: American Society of Clinical Oncology Focused Guideline Update. J Clin Oncol published ahead of print 11.2.15
79. Aapro M, Molassiotis A, Dicato M et al (2012) The effect of guideline-consistent antiemetic therapy on chemotherapy-induced nausea and vomiting (CINV): the Pan European Emesis Registry (PEER). Ann Oncol Off J Eur Soc Med Oncol/ESMO 23(8):1986–1992
80. Gilmore JW, Peacock NW, Gu A et al (2014) Antiemetic guideline consistency and incidence of chemotherapy-induced nausea and vomiting in US community oncology practice: INSPIRE Study. J Oncol Pract/ Am Soc Clin Oncol 10(1):68–74
81. Hesketh P, Aapro M, Jordan K, Schwartzberg L et al (2015) A review of NEPA, a Novel Fixed Antiemetic Combination with the Potential for Enhancing Guideline Adherence and Improving control of chemotherapy-induced nausea and vomiting. Biomed Res Int 2015:651879
82. Calcagnie S, Lanzarotti C, Rossi G et al (2013) Effect of netupitant, a highly selective NK1 receptor antagonist, on the pharmacokinetics of palonesetron and impact of the fixed dose combination of netupitant and palonesetron when coadministered with ketoconazole, rifampicin, and oral contraceptives. Support Care Cancer 21(10):2879–2887
83. Aapro M, Gralla R, Karthaus M et al (2014) Multicycle efficacy and safety of NEPA, a fixed-dose antiemetic combination of netupitant and palonesetron, in patients receiving chemotherapy of varying emetogenicity. Ann Oncol 25 (Suppl 4); IV518-IV519, Abst 1484
84. Hesketh PJ, Rossi G, Rizzi G et al (2014) Efficacy and safety of NEPA, an oral combination of netupitant and palonosetron, for prevention of chemotherapy-induced nausea and vomiting following highly emetogenic chemotherapy: a randomized dose-ranging pivotal study. Ann Oncol Off J Eur Soc Med Oncol/ESMO 25(7):1340–1346
85. Spinelli T, Calcagnile S, Giuliano C et al (2014) Netupitant PET imaging and ADME studies in humans. J Clin Pharmacol 54(1):97–108
86. Aapro M, Rugo H, Rossi G et al (2014) A randomized phase III study evaluating the efficacy and safety of NEPA, a fixed-dose combination of netupitant and palonosetron, for prevention of chemotherapy-induced nausea and vomiting following moderately emetogenic chemotherapy. Ann Oncol Off J Eur Soc Med Oncol/ESMO 25(7):1328–1333
87. Gralla RJ, Bosnjak SM, Hontsa A et al (2014) A phase III study evaluating the safety and efficacy of NEPA, a fixed-dose combination of netupitant and palonosetron, for prevention of chemotherapy-induced nausea and vomiting over repeated cycles of chemotherapy. Ann Oncol Off J Eur Soc Med Oncol/ESMO 25(7):1333–1339
88. Aapro M, Karthaus M, Schwartzberg L et al (2014) Phase 3 study of NEPA, a fixed dose combination of netupitant and palonosetron for prevention of chemotherapy-induced nausea and vomiting during repeated moderately emetogenic chemotherapy (MEC) cycle. J Clin Oncol, 32:5S, Abstract 9502
89. Akynzeo prescribing information (2015) Accessed 12.7.15 www.Akynzeo.com/media/Prescribing_Information.pdf

Chapter 5
The Role of Neurokinin-1 Receptor Antagonists in CINV

Bernardo Leon Rapoport

5.1 Introduction

Significant advances have been made in controlling chemotherapy-induced nausea and vomiting (CINV) in the past two decades. These advances are primarily due to a greater understanding of the physiological and molecular pathways underlying CINV, which resulted in major progress in the management of patients with CINV. In the early 1990s, CINV treatment included dexamethasone [1]. Improvements in the management of CINV control were achieved with the discovery of 5-hydroxytryptamine (5HT3) receptor and the development of 5HT3 receptor antagonists (RA). Additional improvements in CINV control were further made, with the usage of the combination of 5HT3 RA with dexamethasone or other corticosteroid agents at equivalent doses [2, 3].

Over the last decade, the discovery of the neurokinin-1 receptor antagonists (NK1 RA) and its role in the pathogenesis of delayed phase of CINV have led to significant developments in the management of this complication of anticancer treatment. Despite these milestone achievements, nausea and vomiting remain as clinically significant problems for patients undergoing highly emetogenic chemotherapy (HEC) and moderately emetogenic chemotherapy (MEC).

B.L. Rapoport, Dip. in Med., M. Med.
Medical Oncology, The Medical Oncology Center of Rosebank,
129 Oxford Road, Saxonwold, Johannesburg, South Africa
e-mail: brapoport@rosebankoncology.co.za

© Springer International Publishing Switzerland 2016
R.M. Navari (ed.), *Management of Chemotherapy-Induced Nausea and Vomiting: New Agents and New Uses of Current Agents,*
DOI 10.1007/978-3-319-27016-6_5

5.2   MEC- and HEC-Based Chemotherapy

Seventy percent of patients treated with cisplatin-based HEC will achieve an overall antiemetic complete response when managed with a triple therapy consisting of the NK1 RA aprepitant in combination with a 5HT3 RA and corticosteroids prophylaxis [4, 5].

Warr et al. conducted a study in breast cancer women treated with anthracycline and cyclophosphamide (AC)-based moderately emetic chemotherapy (MEC). The study showed that a 3-drug antiemetic regimen with aprepitant had an overall antiemetic complete response rate of 50 %, compared to 42.5 % with a standard two-drug antiemetic regimen without an NK1 RA ($P=0.015$) [6].

Rapoport et al. reported similar outcomes in a comparable MEC patient population with breast cancer [7]. The positive results of these clinical studies have demonstrated the advantage of adding an NK1 RA to antiemetic regimens of 5HT3 RA in combination with corticosteroids and led to its inclusion as an essential component in CINV prophylaxis guidelines [8–10].

5.2.1   Aprepitant and Fosaprepitant

The US Food and Drug Administration (FDA) initially approved aprepitant in 2003 for the treatment of CINV in combination with a 5HT3 RA and dexamethasone. Aprepitant is commonly given as three doses taken orally at a dose of 125 mg before chemotherapy given on day 1 and 80 mg administered on days 2 and 3 [4–6].

Fosaprepitant (a prodrug of aprepitant) is converted to aprepitant via phosphatase enzymes in the bloodstream. Fosaprepitant is an intravenous formulation that can be used in place of the oral dose of aprepitant on day 1. It may be beneficial in patients who cannot tolerate an oral formulation. Fosaprepitant at a dose of 115 mg and oral aprepitant at a dose of 125 mg are bioequivalent and interchangeable. Additionally, a randomized phase III trial conducted by Grunberg et al. has demonstrated non-inferiority between a single-dose intravenous fosaprepitant of 150 mg compared to standard 3-day oral aprepitant (at doses of 125 mg on day 1 and 80 mg on days 2 and 3) for the prevention of CINV during overall and delayed CINV phases [11].

5.2.2   Casopitant

Casopitant was the second NK1 RA undergoing clinical development. A phase III study with casopitant was completed for the treatment of CINV in both 3-day and 1-day dosing schedules. In July 2008, the GlaxoSmithKline (GSK) filed a marketing authorization application to the European Medicines Agency (EMA). GSK decided to withdraw the application in Sep 2009 because the EMA indicated that additional safety evaluation was necessary and that it would take considerable time and resources to produce such data. The potential convenience of dosing the NK1 RA in the clinic without having to prescribe added NK1 doses for patients to take home was of particular interest to the treating clinician as well as patients [12–14].

5.2.3 Netupitant and Rolapitant

Netupitant and rolapitant are other NK1 RA that have been developed for the same indication [15, 16].

Netupitant is being developed in combination with oral palonosetron (NEPA) which was recently registered for the management and prophylaxis of CINV. NEPA consists of a fixed dose of netupitant (a potent and selective NK1 RA) in combination with a fixed dose of palonosetron and targets the two antiemetic pathways [17].

Rolapitant is a third NK1 RA under clinical investigation. This agent is a potent, selective, high-affinity, competitive NK1 receptor antagonist with an extended half-life of approximately 180 h [18].

Positron emission tomography (PET) imaging performed in healthy volunteers 120 h following a single oral 200 mg dose of rolapitant demonstrated a greater than 90 % NK1 receptor occupancy in the brain [19]. The study indicates that a single dose of rolapitant may be sufficient to prevent CINV during the risk period of 0–120 h. Rolapitant is not an inhibitor or inducer of CYP3A4 and is unlikely to have drug–drug interactions with drugs metabolized by CYP3A4, which are utilized for oncology patients undergoing chemotherapy [20]. Consequently, a potential clinical advantage is the fact that fewer drug–drug interactions may not require dose adjustments for concomitant drugs administered with the NK1 receptor antagonist. Dose modifications of anticancer agents could result in a potential loss of efficiency and inferior outcome.

5.3 Clinical Pharmacology of NK1 Inhibitors

Both serotonin (5-HT3) and substance P have been linked in CINV by triggering the corresponding receptors in the brain and the gastrointestinal tissues, respectively [21]. There are substantial differences between substance P and 5-HT3. Substance P and 5-HT3 are thought to have different time courses of action due to the biphasic nature of cisplatin-based HEC (Figs. 5.1 and 5.2) [22, 23]. The 5-HT3-mediated effect occurs within a few hours of the administration of chemotherapy, early in the acute phase. On the other hand, the NK1-mediated effect starts at approximately 15 h following chemotherapy and continues into the delayed phase [23, 24].

While the 5-HT3-mediated phase is short and virtually completed in the first 24 h following chemotherapy administration, the substance P- and NK1-

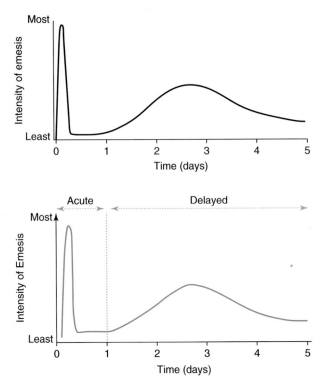

Fig. 5.1 High-dose cisplatin induces an emetogenic biphasic pattern. Tavorath and Hesketh [21]. Martin [26] (Doi:10.1159/000227637)

mediated phase in HEC continues for 60–96 h postchemotherapy [25, 26]. The acute phase of chemotherapy has been arbitrary defined as the initial 24 h post-chemotherapy and the delayed phase as any time in the 96 h after that. These phase definitions are based on the need for readily measurable endpoints, rather than the biological aspects associated with 5-HT3 and NK1. However, the NK1 RA and 5-HT3 RA are often associated with acute and delayed CINV, respectively. It is apparent that the NK1-mediated effect spans both phases in HEC [25, 27].

5.3.1 Aprepitant and Fosaprepitant

AC-based MEC is monophasic, with both the 5-HT3- and NK1-mediated effects occurring within a few hours after chemotherapy, early in the acute phase [23] Fig. 5.2. When the same results were evaluated in patients receiving AC-based MEC, aprepitant was effective beginning in the acute phase, starting as early as 6 h postchemotherapy, compared to approximately 18 h in HEC studies [23, 25].

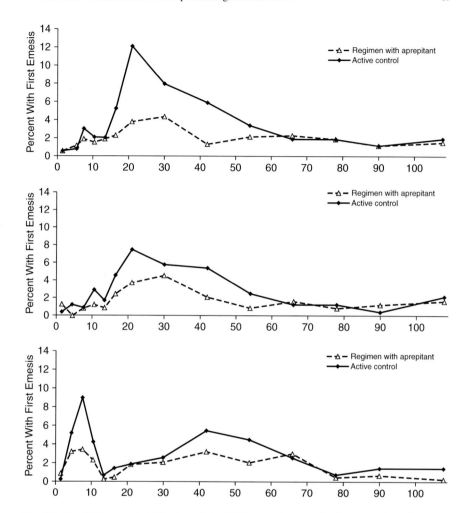

Fig. 5.2 The HEC curve is biphasic and the MEC curve is monophasic. Proportion of patients experiencing first emesis during specified time intervals (0–3, 3–6, 6–9, 9–12, 12–15, 15–18, 18–24, 24–36, 36–48, 48–60, 60–72, 72–84, 84–96, and 96–120 h). *Points* are plotted in the center of each interval. (*Top*) 052/054 studies (cisplatin-based highly emetogenic chemotherapy (HEC). (*Middle*) 071 study (anthracycline plus cyclophosphamide-based MEC). (*Bottom*) 801 study (cisplatin-based HEC)

In cisplatin-based HEC studies, the time to first emesis was evaluated in Kaplan–Meier curves assessing the time to first emesis. The curves depicting the regimen with aprepitant and active control were clearly separated as early as 15 h [23, 25]. Similar effects were observed in NEPA and rolapitant suggesting a class effect of NK1 RA (NEPA and rolapitant in HEC).

The biological variations and the differential time course of action of NK1 RA and 5-HT3 are highlighted when used with HEC and MEC [23, 25]. Although the

NK1 RA are associated fundamentally with the delayed phase, they also have a crucial function through the acute phase in both HEC and MEC as it was noted in the aprepitant studies.

A single dose of oral 125 mg aprepitant has been proved to have a mean plasma half-life of 14.0 h, and at 24 h after dosing, the aprepitant concentration is 36 % of Cmax [27]. The pharmacokinetic profile of aprepitant following administration of intravenous fosaprepitant is similar to that of oral aprepitant. Fosaprepitant is metabolized to active aprepitant following IV administration. The mean plasma half-life of fosaprepitant was found to be 2.3 min, suggesting that the total conversion occurs in less than 30 min [27]. The maximum concentration of aprepitant following IV fosaprepitant administration takes place at 15 min; this is compared to 4 h for aprepitant administered orally. The aprepitant mean half-life was similar for the IV fosaprepitant 115 mg and oral aprepitant 125 mg doses (13.6 h compared to 14.0 h, respectively). These doses had nearly identical mean concentrations at 24 h; 504 ng/mL compared to 494 nanograms/mL, respectively [27].

It is essential to point out that most of the current published NK1 clinical pharmacology literature is with the use of aprepitant. Current clinical studies have investigated the use of netupitant and rolapitant.

5.3.2 Netupitant

Netupitant is an NK1 receptor antagonist with a structure and mechanism of action similar to aprepitant. Netupitant has a high binding affinity with a half-life of 90 h. This agent is metabolized by CYP3A4 and is also an inhibitor of CYP3A4. Netupitant is a moderate inhibitor of the cytochrome P450 3A4 (CYP3A4); a reduction in the oral dexamethasone dose should be considered, when used in conjunction with NEPA [28].

5.3.3 NEPA

NEPA is an oral fixed-dose combination of netupitant and palonosetron. NEPA was recently studied in phase II, and phase III clinical trials for the prevention of CINV in patients getting MEC- and HEC-based treatment. The clinical trials revealed that NEPA (300 mg of netupitant plus 0.50 mg of palonosetron) significantly enhanced the prophylaxis of CINV compared to the use of palonosetron alone in patients undergoing either HEC or MEC [28–30]. Postchemotherapy, there was a significant improvement in the delayed period (24–120 h) and the overall period (0–120 h) with the usage of NEPA. This effect was maintained over multiple cycles of chemotherapy [25].

5.3.4   Rolapitant

Rolapitant is a potent, highly selective, competitive NK1-RA that does not induce or inhibit CYP3A4. The other NK1-RA aprepitant and netupitant do not possess this unique property. The lack of interactions may be an advantage for patients where drug–drug interactions should ideally be avoided.

Rolapitant binds with high affinity (Ki=0·66 nM) to the human NK1 receptor [20] and maintains >90 % receptor binding up to 5 days following a 200 mg dose [19]. Rolapitant also has a long half-life of approximately 180 h [20], indicating that a single dose may be adequate to prevent CINV during the entire 5-day (0–120 h) at-risk period postchemotherapy.

5.4   Clinical Data

5.4.1   Aprepitant

Aprepitant plus ondansetron and dexamethasone was shown to provide significantly greater rates of complete response than ondansetron plus dexamethasone alone in patients receiving cisplatin-based HEC in two phase III trials [4, 5]. Patients were randomized to receive standard therapy with ondansetron (32 mg IV) and dexamethasone (20 mg oral) on day 1 followed by dexamethasone (8 mg bid) on days 2–4. Patients in the aprepitant group received aprepitant (125 mg oral), ondansetron (32 mg IV), and dexamethasone (12 mg oral) on day 1. It was followed by aprepitant (80 mg oral) and dexamethasone (8 mg oral) once daily on days 2, 3 and 4. The first trial evaluated 523 patients for efficacy and 568 patients for safety [5]. The second study assessed 521 patients in the efficacy analysis with 525 patients in the safety analysis [5].

In a joined analysis of these two studies, the complete response rates for the aprepitant group were 86 % compared to the active control group of 73 % for the acute phase. In the delayed phase, it was 72 % versus 51 % and 68 % versus 48 % for the overall 5-day period ($P<0.001$ for all time periods) [25]. In both studies, aprepitant was well tolerated, and the rates of adverse effects and discontinuations were comparable between the two treatment groups [4, 5].

A separate randomized trial compared aprepitant, ondansetron and dexamethasone on day 1; aprepitant and dexamethasone on day 2 and 3, and dexamethasone on day 4 to the control regimen consisting of ondansetron and dexamethasone on days 1 to 4 in patients receiving HEC [31]. The complete response rates for the overall, acute, and delayed were significantly greater in the aprepitant group. In the overall phase (days 1–5), 72 % of the subjects treated with aprepitant had complete response compared to 61 % of patients treated with 4-day ondansetron plus dexamethasone ($P=0.003$) [31].

A special consideration should be given to aprepitant in patients receiving AC-based and non-AC MEC.

In this randomized phase III study, patients undergoing breast cancer chemotherapy were randomly assigned to receive either an aprepitant-containing or an active control regimen for the prevention of CINV ($N=857$). The experimental arm consisted of aprepitant (125 mg) plus ondansetron (8 mg) and dexamethasone (12 mg) on day one of chemotherapy. It was followed by ondansetron (8 mg) 8 h after chemotherapy on day 1, followed by aprepitant at a dose of 80 mg daily on days 2 and 3 [6].

The control group received ondansetron at a dose of 8 mg and dexamethasone at a dose 20 mg prior to chemotherapy, followed by ondansetron 8 mg 8 h later on day 1. Day 2 and day 3 consisted of ondansetron (8 mg bid) [6].

The aprepitant group had a higher complete response rate over the 120 h study duration compared to the control arm (50.8 % versus 42.5 %), respectively; $P=0.015$. A randomized trial conducted by Rapoport et al. assesses the value of aprepitant in MEC regimes (AC and non-AC regimes). This study consisted of a placebo-controlled randomized trial of 848 patients and evaluated the efficacy of the same antiemetic regimen in a range of MEC regimens, including AC-based, oxaliplatin-based, and carboplatin-based chemotherapies [6].

Importantly, in this trial, more patients treated with the aprepitant arm experienced no vomiting (76.2 %) compared to active control (62.1 %; $P<0.001$). These data also demonstrated that antiemetic regimens with aprepitant were also active with other chemotherapy regimens (non-AC) [6].

A separate study examined aprepitant that was administered as a single dose on day 1 in combination with palonosetron and dexamethasone in HEC [31].

This pilot trial consisted of 75 patients who received palonosetron (0.25 mg IV) on day 1 and dexamethasone on days 1–4 [31].

There was no significant variation seen among the single- and 3-day aprepitant dose groups [31]. In both aprepitant cohorts, 93 % of patients were free of emesis during 1 day of follow-up compared with 50 % in the control group [32].

A modification of this aprepitant single-dose protocol in patients receiving MEC was reported in a pilot study with no control group [33]. Forty-one subjects received aprepitant (285 mg oral), dexamethasone (20 mg oral), and palonosetron (0.25 mg IV) given on day 1, with no antiemetics given on subsequent days [33]. In the overall phase, the complete response was 51 %. In the acute phase and the delayed phase, 76 % and 66 % of patients, respectively, attained a complete response consisting of no vomiting or rescue medication usage [33]. This study used a high dose of aprepitant, and no apparent safety concerns emerged during this trial. Although experimental, these studies suggest that aprepitant as a single dose prior to chemotherapy may be feasible.

5.4.2 Casopitant

In phase II trials, casopitant was investigated in various dosing schedules, administered in combination with ondansetron and dexamethasone. Casopitant significantly reduced both HEC- and MEC-associated CINV as measured by the complete response as primary endpoint compared to ondansetron plus dexamethasone alone [12, 13]. These studies included an exploratory single-day regimen of casopitant (150 mg oral). Both the casopitant 3-day IV plus oral and a single oral dose demonstrated efficacy in these trials and were incorporated into the phase III trial design.

The results of these phase III trials of casopitant in HEC have shown that both the single oral dose and the 3-day IV/oral regimen, in combination with ondansetron and dexamethasone (also given on days 2–4), provided significantly improved complete response rates compared with ondansetron and dexamethasone alone: 85.7 % and 79.6 % versus 66.0 % ($P<0.0001$ and $P=0.0004$) [14]. Although casopitant was discontinued for further development, these data provide an important proof of concept to examine the usage of NK1 inhibitors over 1 day. Treatment was well tolerated with similar adverse event and discontinuation frequency across study arms [14].

5.4.3 Fosaprepitant

The bioequivalence of intravenous fosaprepitant 115 mg to oral aprepitant 125 mg was confirmed in a 3-part randomized pharmacokinetic study in healthy adult volunteers [34].

Single-day one dosing of fosaprepitant for HEC was studied in phase III [11–36]. Grunberg et al. conducted a randomized, double-blind, active control design to test non-inferiority between fosaprepitant and aprepitant. HEC-naïve patients treated with cisplatin at a dose equal or greater than 70 mg/m^2 got ondansetron and dexamethasone and a standard aprepitant regimen of 125 mg on day 1, 80 mg on day 2, 80 mg on day 3, compared to a single-dose fosaprepitant regimen of 150 mg on day 1. The primary endpoint of the study was CR (defined as no vomiting, no rescue medication during the overall phase). The study enrolled a total of 2,322 patients; a total of 2,247 were evaluable for efficacy. These data confirm that antiemetic protection with aprepitant and fosaprepitant was non-inferior. More frequent infusion site pain, erythema, and thrombophlebitis were seen with fosaprepitant compared to aprepitant (2.7 % vs. 0.3 %, respectively).

In a separate study, Saito et al. [35] assessed the effectiveness and safety of single-dose fosaprepitant in combination with intravenous granisetron and dexamethasone in patients receiving cisplatin-based HEC chemotherapy at doses ≥70 mg/m^2. In total, 347 patients were entered to receive the fosaprepitant 150 mg on day 1 in combination with granisetron 40 μg/kg and dexamethasone. All drugs were given intravenously. The control regimen consisted of placebo plus intravenous granisetron and dexamethasone. The percentage of patients who attained a CR was significantly greater in the fosaprepitant group than in the control group (64 % compared to 47 %, $P=0.0015$). The fosaprepitant regimen was more active than the control treatment in the acute phase (94 % vs. 81 %, $P=0.0006$) as well as the delayed phase (65 % vs. 49 %, $P=0.0025$). These authors concluded that a single-dose fosaprepitant given in combination with granisetron and dexamethasone was well tolerated and active in preventing CINV in patients treated with HEC. This study shows that a single dose of aprepitant or fosaprepitant also improves the antiemetic effects provided by standard 5HT3 RA and corticosteroid therapy over standard therapy alone. It also provides a comparable level of efficacy as a 3-day aprepitant regimen.

5.4.4 Dosing Over Multiple Chemotherapy Cycles

The efficacy of aprepitant in protecting against CINV experienced over multiple cycles of cisplatin-based chemotherapy was reported in two different studies [36, 37]. One of these studies evaluated extension data from the two large randomized phase III clinical trials, evaluating the protective efficacy of aprepitant against CINV over additional multiple courses of chemotherapy treatment. A total of 1,099 patients from these phase III studies continued receiving the same antiemetic agents they had been using for up to five additional cycles of chemotherapy [37]. The trial was designed to investigate a combined exploratory endpoint of no emesis and no significant nausea (defined as nausea interfering with a patient's normal activities). The aprepitant control rates over the multiple cycles were consistently higher than those in the group receiving standard therapy ($P \leq 0.006$ for all cycles) [37]. The rate of CINV prophylaxis showed a minimal loss of protection from cycle 1 to cycle 6, indicating that antiemetic effects of aprepitant are sustained through multiple cycles of chemotherapy [37]. Also, aprepitant was well tolerated with repeated dosing [37].

5.4.5 Rolapitant

Rolapitant is a promising agent and was studied in multicenter, randomized, double-blind, placebo-controlled, dose range-finding study given orally in subjects receiving highly emetogenic chemotherapy (HEC ≥ 70 mg/m^2 cisplatin-based chemotherapy). The study included a total of 454 subjects. Patients were randomized to receive ondansetron, dexamethasone, and either placebo of 10, 25, 100, or 200 mg of rolapitant prior to treatment with cisplatin on day 1 of each cycle. The rolapitant 200 mg group had significantly greater CR in the overall, acute phase and delayed phase when compared to the control group (62.5 % vs. 46.7 %, $p=0.032$; 87.6 % vs. 66.7 %, $p=0.001$; and 63.6 % vs. 48.9 %, $p=0.045$) [38].

Of interest these patients had higher rates of no significant nausea (a maximum visual analog score <25 mm) in the overall, acute, and delayed phases compared to the control group (63.2 % vs. 42.2 %, $p=0.005$; 86.5 % vs. 73.3 %, $p=0.029$; and 64.4 % vs. 47.8 %, $p=0.026$, respectively). These results suggested a benefit over current treatments. Nausea continues to be a clinically significant problem in the management of CINV. These findings were recently confirmed in two randomized phase III studies with adequate design and validated endpoints (Rapoport ASCO

2014) [39, 40]). This phase III program comprised of two global, randomized, double-blind, active-controlled, parallel-group phase III studies. Patients received an oral 180-mg rolapitant dose or placebo before HEC administration (rolapitant HEC-1 study with 526; rolapitant HEC-2 study, with 544 patients). All patients received granisetron (10 µg/kg intravenously) and dexamethasone (20 mg orally) on day 1 and dexamethasone (8 mg orally) on days 2–4. The primary endpoint was complete response (CR) rate (no emesis or rescue medication) in the delayed phase (>24–120 h). The two rolapitant HEC studies achieved the primary endpoint, and rolapitant demonstrated superiority over the active control. Rolapitant-treated patients had significantly higher CR rates (odds ratio [95 % CI]) than controls in the delayed phase (HEC-1 ($72 \cdot 7$ % vs. $58 \cdot 4$ %) and HEC-2 ($70 \cdot 1$ % vs. $61 \cdot 9$ %); pooled studies, $71 \cdot 4$ % vs. $60 \cdot 2$ %)[39].

The MEC program consisted of a global, randomized, double-blind, active-controlled, parallel-group phase III study of 1,344 patient naïve to MEC or HEC. Patients were randomized to receive a 180-mg rolapitant single dose or placebo approximately 30 min prior to an administration of MEC. Approximately half of those patients received anthracycline/cyclophosphamide (AC)-based chemotherapy (703 patients) and the other half non-AC chemotherapy (629 patients).

The primary endpoint of the MEC study was complete response rate consisting of no emesis or rescue medication in the delayed phase (>24–120 h).

This MEC study successfully achieved the primary endpoint. Treatment with rolapitant resulted in a significantly higher CR rate in the delayed phase ($71 \cdot 3$ % vs. $61 \cdot 6$ %, $p < 0 \cdot 001$) compared with control. The trial demonstrated the advantage of adding an NK1 RA to active control for the prevention of CINV in patients receiving MEC. A prespecified exploratory logistic regression analysis, which adjusted for gender, region, age, and use of AC-based chemotherapy confirmed the primary analysis. When analyzed by chemotherapy subgroups for both AC-based (66.9 % vs. 59.5; $p = 0.05$) and non-AC-based (76.1 % vs. $63 \cdot 8$; $p = <0.001$) subgroups, treatment with rolapitant resulted in significantly higher CR rates than control in the delayed phase in both subgroups.

5.4.6 Netupitant

NEPA is an oral fixed-dose combination of netupitant and palonosetron. The combination targets the two pathways associated with acute and delayed CINV, the serotonin and the substance P-mediated pathways. NEPA was researched in recent phase II and phase III clinical trials for the prophylaxis of CINV in patients receiving MEC and HEC regimes.

A different characteristic of palonosetron is related to the binding of the 5-HT3 receptor and is markedly different from the binding of the ondansetron, granisetron, tropisetron, and dolasetron [41, 42]. The binding property is possibly improving the effects in the delayed CINV compared to the first-generation 5-HT3 receptor antagonists.

A recent phase III, multinational, randomized, double-blind, parallel-group study evaluated the efficacy and safety of a single oral dose of NEPA (netupitant 300 mg and palonosetron 0.50 mg) compared to a single oral 0.50 mg dose of palonosetron as a single agent. A total of 1,455 chemotherapy-naïve patients receiving anthracycline-based chemotherapy were enrolled into the study. All patients received oral dexamethasone at a dose of 12 mg in the NEPA arm, or 20 mg of dexamethasone in the palonosetron arm, on the first day of each cycle.

Most patients were white females undergoing treatment for breast cancer. The primary endpoint of the trial was CR during the delayed phase (25–120 h). NEPA showed superiority in terms of CR rates compared to palonosetron during the delayed, acute, and overall phases. NEPA was also better to palonosetron during the delayed and overall phases for complete protection defined as no emesis and no significant nausea. Treatment with NEPA was well tolerated. The frequency of headache was 3.3 % and constipation 2.1 %. The authors concluded that NEPA was superior to palonosetron in preventing CINV in breast cancer patients receiving MEC. Additionally, there was no evidence of any cardiac safety concerns for NEPA or palonosetron [28].

In summary, dexamethasone doses in the NEPA trials were 12 mg orally on day 1 (for HEC/AC). An additional 8 mg on days 2–4 in the HEC setting should be administered. For patients receiving HEC and MEC, the dexamethasone doses to be prescribed with NEPA are similar to the dose recommended for aprepitant.

5.5   NEPA in HEC and MEC

NEPA was also assessed in HEC. The first was a double-blind, parallel-group trial in 694 chemotherapy naïve patients undergoing cisplatin-based HEC chemotherapy. The study compared three different doses of oral netupitant 100, 200 and 300 mg plus palonosetron 0,5 mg (NEPA) to oral palonosetron 0.5 mg given on day 1. An additional comparator control arm consisted of a standard 3-day oral aprepitant and IV ondansetron at a dose of 32 mg regimen. Patients in all treatment arms got oral dexamethasone on days 1 to day 4 [28]. The primary efficacy endpoint was the complete response for the overall (0–120 h) phase.

Results of this study showed that all the NEPA arms of the study were significantly superior in terms of overall complete response rates compared to palonosetron alone. The 300-mg NEPA dose showed a numerical improvement over the lower doses. Additionally, there was no significant difference detected in the overall complete response in the NEPA treatment arms and the aprepitant arm. NEPA had a low incidence of adverse events in all treatment groups [28].

A phase III clinical trial was conducted for the prevention of CINV in patients receiving MEC [43]. The study was a multinational, randomized, double-blind, parallel-group phase III trial in 1,455 chemotherapy naïve patients receiving MEC (patients receiving anthracycline and cyclophosphamide were included in the trial). Patients were randomized to a single oral dose of NEPA at a dose of 300-mg netupitant with palonosetron at a dose of 0.50 mg or a single oral dose of palonosetron (0.50 mg) prior to the administration of chemotherapy on day 1. All patients received oral dexamethasone on day 1 at a dose of 12 mg in the NEPA arm or 20 mg of dexamethasone in the palonosetron arm. The primary efficacy endpoint was the complete response during the delayed (24–120 h) time. The complete response during the delayed phase was significantly superior to the NEPA group of patients compared to the palonosetron patient group. NEPA had a good tolerability and a similar side effect profile compared to palonosetron [43].

5.6   NEPA in Subsequent Cycles of Chemotherapy

A multiple cycle extension study was conducted in of 1,286 patients of the original 1,455 patients in the MEC phase III trial. Four cycles of chemotherapy were completed in 76 % of the patients. Treatment groups were comparable. NEPA group superiority was proved compared to the palonosetron group for complete response in the overall (0–120 h) period in cycle one that was shown during the multiple cycles of chemotherapy. Patients receiving NEPA had a low incidence of adverse events, consisting of headache in 3.5 % and constipation in 2.0 %, during the multiple cycle extension. There was no difference in adverse reactions in the NEPA compared to the palonosetron group [25].

NEPA appears to be associated with a better control of nausea compared to palonosetron alone. The patients treated in two randomized, multinational studies [28, 43] who underwent NEPA (fixed dose of netupitant 300 mg plus palonosetron 0.50 mg) or palonosetron and dexamethasone prior to chemotherapy treatment with cisplatin or anthracycline plus cyclophosphamide were evaluated for no significant nausea (<25 mm, 0–100 mm, visual analog scale). The NEPA group had a higher number of patients with no significant nausea; this effect was most manifest in the delayed nausea phase of the cisplatin group of patients [44].

The US FDA approved NEPA (Akynzeo®, Helsinn Healthcare SA, Switzerland) to treat chemotherapy-induced nausea and vomiting in October 2014 [45].

5.7   NK1 RA with High-Dose Chemotherapy and in Peripheral Stem Cell Transplantation

5.7.1   Aprepitant

Highly emetogenic preparative regimens before autologous or allogeneic SCT typically take up to a week to administer; therefore, the need to deliver aprepitant for longer than the 3 days approved by the FDA might have safety implications. A recent randomized phase III study investigating the use of antiemetic regimen administered on each day of the preparative regimen plus an additional 1–3 days has recently been reported. The clinical study tested ondansetron and dexamethasone with or without aprepitant in 264 patients that have been treated with high-dose preparatory regimens and showed a significant reduction in emesis and nausea, without increasing regimen-related toxicity or the use of rescue medication [46].

A similar study, assessing the combination of aprepitant, palonosetron, and dexamethasone, revealed that the combination was safe and efficacious for the prevention of nausea and emesis in patients receiving high-dose BEAM (carmustine, etoposide, cytarabine, melphalan) prior to hematopoietic SCT [47]. Furthermore, an aprepitant-based antiemetic regimen given prior to high-dose cytarabine showed a minimal effect on autologous peripheral blood stem cell mobilization [48].

Aprepitant did not alter the pharmacokinetics of high-dose melphalan used as conditioning therapy before SCT in patients with multiple myeloma [49].

The efficacy of aprepitant in patients with multiple myeloma undergoing chemotherapy with autologous stem cell transplant was investigated in two phase II [50, 51] and one phase III clinical studies [50]. The phase II studies are difficult to evaluate because these small studies have different response and eligibility criteria [50, 51]. A phase III study was recently published. Eligible patients with multiple myeloma were randomized to receive either aprepitant administered at a dose of 125 mg orally on day 1 and 80 mg orally on days 2–4, granisetron (at a dose of 2 mg orally on days 1–4), and dexamethasone (at a dose of 4 mg orally on day 1 and 2 mg orally on days 2–3) or matching placebo. The placebo arm consisted of granisetron (at a dose of 2 mg orally on days 1–4) and dexamethasone (at a dose of 8 mg orally on day 1 and 4 mg orally on days 2–3). The high-dose chemotherapy consisted of melphalan at a dose of 100 mg/m^2 was administered intravenously on days 1–2. The autologous stem cell translation was performed on day 4. The primary endpoint was a complete response, defined as no emesis and no rescue therapy within 120 h of melphalan administration [50].

A total of 362 patients were available for the efficacy analysis, with 181 in each treatment arm. Patients who attained a complete response were significantly higher in the aprepitant arm compared to the control group (58 % vs. 41 %; 95 % CI, 1.23–3.00; $P=0.0042$). Absence of major nausea (94 % vs. 88 %; CI, 1.09–5.15; $P=0.026$) and emesis (78 % vs. 65 %; 95 % CI, 1.25–3.18; $P=0.0036$) within 120 h was significantly increased by aprepitant. The mean total FLIE score (± standard deviation) was 114 ± 18 for aprepitant and 106 ± 26 for placebo ($P<0.001$).

The authors concluded that the addition of aprepitant resulted in significantly less CINV and had a positive impact on the quality of life, in patients with multiple myeloma undergoing high-dose melphalan and stem cell rescue [50]. Aprepitant was well tolerated in the three multiple myeloma studies [50].

It is important to emphasize that until recently there are very few studies assessing the efficient use of antiemetics for patients undergoing high-dose chemotherapy with stem cell support. Most reports include phase II investigations of a 5-HT3 receptor antagonist alone or in combination with dexamethasone. A major challenge in evaluating patients in this setting is the multifactorial nature of nausea and vomiting in this setting. In addition to chemotherapy agents, other contributing causes of emesis include the use of antibiotics administered prophylactically, narcotic analgesics, and in some patients the usage of total body irradiation. Cross comparison of studies is complicated due to the varied chemotherapy regimens and different patient populations and tumor types. Additionally, the majority of patients have experienced emesis with prior chemotherapy or irradiation.

5.7.2 Adverse Events Related to NK1 RA

The incidence of toxicities of NK1 RA was assessed in a systematic review of 17 trials with 8,740 patients when NK1 RA are added to 5HT RA and corticosteroids antiemetic regimens for the prevention of CINV. It was noted that the addition of an NK1 RA resulted in a statistically significant, but clinically trivial, differences in fatigue and hiccups compared with controls [52]. The study also demonstrated a statistically significant increase in the risk of severe infection among patients who received NK1 RA (OR 3.10; $P < 0.001$) [52]. It is important to highlight that the difference was largely from an individual study, which used high doses of dexamethasone [53] and not primarily from the use of aprepitant.

Fosaprepitant has similar tolerability profile to aprepitant. However, fosaprepitant is associated with a higher incidence of infusion site adverse events (2.2 % vs. 0.4 %) and significantly more thrombophlebitis (0.8 %. vs. 0.1 %; $P = 0.005$) [54].

5.7.3 Drug–Drug Interactions with NK1 RA

Aprepitant is extensively metabolized by liver enzymes, primarily CYP3A4; therefore, potent CYP3A4 inhibitors can increase aprepitant exposure, and potent CYP3A4 inducers can reduce aprepitant exposure [55]. Aprepitant is also, paradoxically, both an inducer and a moderate inhibitor of CYP3A4 [56]. Thus, the potential for drug–drug interactions exists when aprepitant is coadministered with other drugs that are metabolized by CYP enzymes, including chemotherapeutic agents [57].

Netupitant is metabolized by CYP3A4 and is also an inhibitor of CYP3A4. Netupitant is a moderate inhibitor of the cytochrome P450 3A4 (CYP3A4). Therefore, drug-drug interactions are possible, similar to aprepitant.

Rolapitant is a potent, highly selective, competitive NK1 RA. It does not induce or inhibit CYP3A4. The other NK1 RA aprepitant and netupitant does not possess this unique property. This unique mechanism of action may be usual in patients with comorbidities requiring concurrent medications.

5.8 Future Directions and Current Guidelines

Multinational Association of Supportive Care in Cancer (MASCC), the National Comprehensive Cancer Network (NCCN), and the American Society for Clinical Oncology (ASCO) have developed evidence-based guidelines.

Evidence-based indications for the usage of NK1 RA are endorsed in combination with 5-HT3 RA and dexamethasone (triple therapy prophylaxis). Triple therapy is recommended as the preferred treatment for preventing CINV associated with HEC and MEC AC-based chemotherapy.

Fosaprepitant was recently evaluated in non-AC in a global, phase III, randomized, double-blind trial. The study included naïve to MEC and HEC patients. Subjects were randomly assigned 1:1 to a control or fosaprepitant regimen. The control group received treatment with oral ondansetron at a dose of 8 mg, 20 mg of dexamethasone, and IV saline as placebo before the first dose of MEC on day 1 and 8 mg of oral ondansetron 8 h after the first dose, followed by 8 mg of oral ondansetron every 12 h on days 2 and 3. Patients in the fosaprepitant regimen received the similar dose of oral ondansetron on day 1, along with 12-mg dexamethasone and a single dose of 150-mg IV fosaprepitant before the first dose of MEC on day 1, with no additional prophylactic antiemetic beyond day 1. The study population consisted of 1,000 patients (502 received fosaprepitant and 498 in the control group). In the study, the primary endpoint was CR during the delayed phase. The study achieved the primary endpoint. CR in the delayed phase was achieved in 396 patients (78.9 %) in the fosaprepitant arm and 341 patients (68.5 %) in the control arm during the delayed phase (treatment difference of 10.4 %, $P < 0.001$) [58].

The recent fosaprepitant and the rolapitant MEC study are potentially practice-changing [28, 36–52]. It is very likely that these studies will result in the guideline inclusion of NK1 RA for the prophylaxis of non-AC MEC regimes including carboplatin and non-carboplatin non-AC-based treatments.

Another important indication for guideline inclusion is the usage of NK1 RA for the prevention of CINV in patients undergoing high-dose chemotherapy and stem cell support. Recent phase III studies demonstrate the beneficial effect of NK1 RA in this indication.

Finally, an additional indication for triple antiemetic prophylaxis for CINV includes patients with germ cell tumors undergoing multiple-day cis-platinum-based treatment. Aprepitant in this setting was studied in 71 patients' randomized trial. Among 69 patients were evaluable, and 35 patients were randomly assigned to receive an aprepitant-based triple therapy antiemetic prophylaxis and 34 to receive placebo, 5HT3 RA and corticosteroids antiemetic prophylaxis for the first course of chemotherapy treatment. The study showed that 42 % achieved a CR with aprepitant compared with 13 % with placebo ($P < 0.001$). Eleven patients (16.2 %) had at least one emetic episode during the aprepitant cycle versus 32 patients (47.1 %) with placebo. There was no additional toxicity with aprepitant compared with placebo [59].

5.9 Conclusion

Antiemetic therapy has advanced significantly in the last decade with the addition of NK1 RA to the therapeutic options. Aprepitant, fosaprepitant, netupitant, and rolapitant enhance the effectiveness of the antiemetic combination of a corticosteroid and 5HT3 RA for controlling the acute and delayed phases of CINV. There has been a significant improvement in CR rate with aprepitant combined with a 5HT3-RA and dexamethasone for patients undergoing HEC, AC, and MEC non-AC regimes. Additionally, the use of aprepitant was associated with an improvement in CR in patients undergoing high-dose chemotherapy with stem cell support and patients undergoing multiple-day chemotherapy treatments. These new developments are likely to be reflected in CINV guidelines soon.

References

1. Aapro MS, Alberts DS (1981) Dexamethasone as an antiemetic in patients treated with cisplatin. N Engl J Med 305(9):520
2. Falkson G, van Zyl AJ (1989) A phase I study of a new 5HT3-receptor antagonist, BRL43694A, an agent for the prevention of chemotherapy-induced nausea and vomiting. Cancer Chemother Pharmacol 24(3):193–196
3. Smith DB, Newlands ES, Spruyt OW, Begent RH, Rustin GJ, Mellor B, Bagshawe KD (1990) Ondansetron (GR38032F) plus dexamethasone: effective anti-emetic prophylaxis for patients receiving cytotoxic chemotherapy. Br J Cancer 61(2):323–324
4. Hesketh PJ, Grunberg SM, Gralla RJ et al (2003) The oral neurokinin-1 antagonist aprepitant for the prevention of chemotherapy-induced nausea and vomiting: a multinational, randomized, double-blind, placebo-controlled trial in patients receiving high-dose cisplatin--the aprepitant protocol 052 study group. J Clin Oncol 21:4112–4119
5. Poli-Bigelli S, Rodrigues-Pereira J, Carides AD et al (2003) Addition of the neurokinin 1 receptor antagonist aprepitant to standard antiemetic therapy improves control of chemotherapy-induced nausea and vomiting. Results from a randomized, double-blind, placebo-controlled trial in Latin America. Cancer 97:3090–3098
6. Warr DG, Hesketh PJ, Gralla RJ et al (2005) Efficacy and tolerability of aprepitant for the prevention of chemotherapy-induced nausea and vomiting in patients with breast cancer after moderately emetogenic chemotherapy. J Clin Oncol 23:2822–2830
7. Rapoport BL, Jordan K, Boice JA, et al (2010) Aprepitant for the prevention of chemotherapy-induced nausea and vomiting associated with a broad range of moderately emetogenic chemotherapies and tumor types: a randomized, double-blind study. Support Care Cancer 18(14):428–431
8. National Comprehensive Cancer Network. NCNN Guidelines 1.2012: Antiemesis 1.2012. 2012. Report No.: 1.2012
9. Roila F, Herrstedt J, Aapro M et al (2010) Guideline update for MASCC and ESMO in the prevention of chemotherapy- and radiotherapy-induced nausea and vomiting: results of the Perugia consensus conference. Ann Oncol 21(Suppl 5):v232–v243
10. Hesketh PJ, Bohlke K, Lyman GH, Basch E, Chesney M, Clark-Snow RA, Danso MA, Jordan K, Somerfield MR, Kris MG. Antiemetics: American Society of Clinical Oncology Focused Guideline Update. J Clin Oncol. 2015 Nov 2. pii: JCO.2015.64.3635. [Epub ahead of print]
11. Grunberg S, Chua D, Maru A, Dinis J, DeVandry S, Boice JA, Hardwick JS, Beckford E, Taylor A, Carides A, Roila F, Herrstedt J (2011) Single-dose fosaprepitant for the prevention

of chemotherapy-induced nausea and vomiting associated with cisplatin therapy: randomized, double-blind study protocol--EASE. J Clin Oncol 29(11):1495–1501

12. Arpornwirat W, Albert I, Hansen VL et al (2009) Phase 2 trial results with the novel neuroki- nin-1 receptor antagonist casopitant in combination with ondansetron and dexamethasone for the prevention of chemotherapy-induced nausea and vomiting in cancer patients receiving moderately emetogenic chemotherapy. Cancer 115(24):5807–5816

13. Roila F, Rolski J, Ramlau R et al (2009) Randomized, double-blind, dose-ranging trial of the oral neurokinin-1 receptor antagonist casopitant mesylate for the prevention of cisplatin- induced nausea and vomiting. Ann Oncol 20(11):1867–1873

14. Grunberg SM, Rolski J, Strausz J et al (2009) Efficacy and safety of casopitant mesylate, a neurokinin 1 (NK_1)-receptor antagonist, in prevention of chemotherapy-induced nausea and vomiting in patients receiving cisplatin-based highly emetogenic chemotherapy: a randomised, double-blind, placebo-controlled trial. Lancet Oncol 10:549–558

15. Stathis M, Pietra C, Rojas C, Slusher BS (2012) Inhibition of substance P-mediated responses in NG108-15 cells by netupitant and palonosetron exhibit synergistic effects. Eur J Pharmacol 689(1-3):25–30

16. Duffy RA, Morgan C, Naylor R, Higgins GA, Varty GB, Lachowicz JE, Parker EM (2012) Rolapitant (SCH 619734): a potent, selective and orally active neurokinin NK1 receptor antag- onist with centrally-mediated antiemetic effects in ferrets. Pharmacol Biochem Behav 102(1):95–100

17. Calcagnile S, Lanzarotti C, Rossi G, Henriksson A, Kammerer KP, Timmer W (2013) Effect of netupitant, a highly selective NK_1 receptor antagonist, on the pharmacokinetics of palono- setron and impact of the fixed dose combination of netupitant and palonosetron when coad- ministered with ketoconazole, rifampicin, and oral contraceptives. Support Care Cancer 21(10):2879–2887

18. Gan TJ, Gu J, Singla N, Chung F, Pearman MH, Bergese SD, Habib AS, Candiotti KA, Mo Y, Huyck S, Creed MR, Cantillon M, Rolapitant Investigation Group (2011) Rolapitant for the prevention of postoperative nausea and vomiting: a prospective, double-blinded, placebo- controlled randomized trial. Anesth Analg 112(4):804–812

19. Poma A, Christensen J, Davis J, Kansra V, Martell RE, Hedley ML. Phase 1 positron emission tomography (PET) study of the receptor occupancy of rolapitant, a novel NK-1 receptor antag- onist. J Clin Oncol 2014; 32(suppl):abstr e20690

20. Poma A, Christensen J, Pentikis H et al (2013) Rolapitant and its major metabolite do not affect the pharmacokinetics of midazolam, a sensitive cytochrome P450 3A4 Substrate. Abstract 0441, MASCC/ISOO Symposium 2013. Support Care Cancer 21(1 Suppl)

21. Tavorath R, Hesketh PJ (1996) Drug treatment of chemotherapy-induced delayed emesis. Drugs 52:639–648

22. Wilder-Smith OH, Borgeat A, Chappuis P et al (1993) Urinary serotonin metabolite excretion during cisplatin chemotherapy. Cancer 72:2239–2241

23. Hesketh PJ, Warr DG, Street JC et al (2011) Differential time course of action of 5-HT3 and NK1 receptor antagonists when used with highly and moderately emetogenic chemotherapy (HEC and MEC). Support Care Cancer 19(9):1297–1302

24. Mantovani G, Maccio A, Curreli L et al (1998) Comparison of oral 5-HT_3-receptor antago- nists and low-dose oral metoclopramide plus I.M. dexamethasone for the prevention of delayed emesis in head and neck cancer patients receiving high-dose cisplatin. Oncol Rep 5:273–280

25. Warr DG, Grunberg SM, Gralla RJ et al (2005) The oral NK(1) antagonist aprepitant for the prevention of acute and delayed chemotherapy-induced nausea and vomiting: pooled data from 2 randomised, double-blind, placebo controlled trials. Eur J Cancer 41:1278–1285

26. Martin M (1996) The severity and pattern of emesis following different cytotoxic agents. Oncology 53(Suppl 1):26–31

27. Lasseter KC, Gambale J, Jin B et al (2007) Tolerability of fosaprepitant and bioequivalency to aprepitant in healthy subjects. J Clin Pharmacol 47:834–840

28. Hesketh PJ, Rossi G, Rizzi G, Palmas M, Alyasova A, Bondarenko I, Lisyanskaya A, Gralla RJ (2014) Efficacy and safety of NEPA, an oral combination of netupitant and palonosetron,

for prevention of chemotherapy-induced nausea and vomiting following highly emetogenic chemotherapy: a randomized dose-ranging pivotal study. Ann Oncol 25(7):1340–1346

29. Rapoport BL, Poma A, Hedley ML et al (2014) Phase 3 trial results for rolapitant, a novel NK-1 receptor antagonist, in the prevention of chemotherapy-induced nausea and vomiting (CINV) in subjects receiving highly emetogenic chemotherapy (HEC). J Clin Oncol 32:32

30. Aapro M, Karthaus M, Schwartzberg LS et al (2014) Phase 3 study of NEPA, a fixed-dose combination of netupitant and palonosetron, for prevention of chemotherapy-induced nausea and vomiting during repeated moderately emetogenic chemotherapy cycles [abstract]. J Clin Oncol 32(Suppl 5):9502

31. Schmoll HJ, Aapro MS, Poli-Bigelli S, Kim HK, Park K, Jordan K, von Pawel J, Giezek H, Ahmed T, Chan CY (2006) Comparison of an aprepitant regimen with a multiple-day ondansetron regimen, both with dexamethasone, for antiemetic efficacy in high-dose cisplatin treatment. Ann Oncol 17(6):1000–1006

32. Herrington JD, Jaskiewicz AD, Song J (2008) Randomized, placebo-controlled, pilot study evaluating aprepitant single dose plus palonosetron and dexamethasone for the prevention of acute and delayed chemotherapy-induced nausea and vomiting. Cancer 112:2080–2087.24

33. Grunberg SM, Dugan M, Muss H et al (2009) Effectiveness of a single-day three-drug regimen of dexamethasone, palonosetron, and aprepitant for the prevention of acute and delayed nausea and vomiting caused by moderately emetogenic chemotherapy. Support Care Cancer 17:589–594

34. Van Belle SJ, Cocquyt V (2008) Fosaprepitant dimeglumine (MK-0517 or L-785,298), an intravenous neurokinin-1 antagonist for the prevention of chemotherapy induced nausea and vomiting. Expert Opin Pharmacother 9(18):3261–3270

35. Saito H, Yoshizawa H, Yoshimori K, Katakami N, Katsumata N, Kawahara M, Eguchi K (2013) Efficacy and safety of single-dose fosaprepitant in the prevention of chemotherapy-induced nausea and vomiting in patients receiving high-dose cisplatin: a multicentre, randomised, double-blind, placebo-controlled phase 3 trial. Ann Oncol 24(4):1067–1073

36. de Wit R, Herrstedt J, Rapoport B, Carides AD, Guoguang-Ma J, Elmer M, Schmidt C, Evans JK, Horgan KJ (2004) The oral NK(1) antagonist, aprepitant, given with standard antiemetics provides protection against nausea and vomiting over multiple cycles of cisplatin-based chemotherapy: a combined analysis of two randomised, placebo-controlled phase III clinical trials. Eur J Cancer 40(3):403–410

37. de Wit R, Herrstedt J, Rapoport B, Carides AD, Carides G, Elmer M, Schmidt C, Evans JK, Horgan KJ (2003) Addition of the oral NK1 antagonist aprepitant to standard antiemetics provides protection against nausea and vomiting during multiple cycles of cisplatin-based chemotherapy. J Clin Oncol 21(22):4105–4111

38. Rapoport B, Chua D, Poma A, Arora S, Wang Y, Fein LE (2015) Study of rolapitant, a novel, long-acting, NK-1 receptor antagonist, for the prevention of chemotherapy-induced nausea and vomiting (CINV) due to highly emetogenic chemotherapy (HEC). Support Care Cancer 23(11):3281–3288

39. Rapoport BL, Poma A, Hedley ML, Martel RE, Navari RM (2014) Phase III trial results for rolapitant, a novel NK-1 receptor antagonist, in the prevention of chemotherapy-induced nausea and vomiting (CINV) in subjects receiving highly emetogenic chemotherapy (HEC) [abstract] J Clin Oncol 32(Suppl 5):9638. Rapoport B, Chasen M, Gridelli M, Urban L, Modiano M, Schnadig I, Poma A, Arora S, Kansra V, Schwartzberg L, Navari R Safety and efficacy assessment of rolapitant for the prevention of chemotherapy-induced nausea and vomiting following administration of cisplatin-based highly emetogenic chemotherapy in cancer patients in two randomised Phase 3 Trials. Lancet Oncol (Manuscript in press)

40. Schnadig ID, Modiano MR, Poma A, Hedley ML, Martel RE, Schwartzberg LS (2014) Phase III trial results for rolapitant, a novel NK-1 receptor antagonist, in the prevention of chemotherapy-induced nausea and vomiting (CINV) in subjects receiving moderately emetogenic chemotherapy (MEC) [abstract] J Clin Oncol 32(Suppl 5):9633. Schwartzberg L, Modiano M, Rapoport B, Chasen M, Gridelli B, Urban L, Poma A, Arora S, Navari R, Schnadig I Safety and efficacy assessment of rolapitant for the prevention of chemotherapy-induced nausea and vomiting following administration of moderately emetogenic chemotherapy in cancer patients in a randomised phase 3 trial. Lancet Oncol (Manuscript in press)

41. Rojas C, Thomas AG, Alt J et al (2010) Palonosetron triggers 5-HT3 receptor internalization and causes prolonged inhibition of receptor function. Eur J Pharmacol 626:193–199
42. Rojas C, Slusher BS (2012) Pharmacological mechanisms of 5-HT3 tachykinin NK-1 receptor antagonism to prevent chemotherapy-induced nausea and vomiting. Eur J Pharmacol 684:1–7
43. Aapro M, Rugo H, Rossi G et al (2014) A randomized phase III study evaluating the efficacy and safety of NEPA, a fixed-dose combination of netupitant and palonosetron, for prevention of chemotherapy-induced nausea and vomiting following moderately emetogenic chemotherapy. Ann Oncol 25:1328–1333
44. Schwartzberg L, Aapro M, Hesketh PJ et al (2014) do NK-1 receptor antagonists contribute to nausea control. Evaluation of the novel NEPA fixed-dose combination of NK-1 receptor antagonist plus a 5-HT3 receptor antagonist from pivotal trials. Support Care Cancer 22:S107, Abstract 161
45. US Food and Drug Administration (2014) FDA approves Akynzeo for nausea and vomiting associated with cancer chemotherapy [press release]. US Food and Drug Administration, Silver Springs, Accessed 30 Apr 2015. Available from: http://www.fda.gov/NewsEvents/Newsroom/PressAnnouncements
46. Stiff PJ, Fox-Geiman MP, Kiley K et al (2013) Prevention of nausea and vomiting associated with stem cell transplant: results of a prospective, randomized trial of aprepitant used with highly emetogenic preparative regimens. Biol Blood Marrow Transplant 19(1):49–55
47. Pielichowski W, Barzal J, Gawronski K et al (2011) A triple-drug combination to prevent nausea and vomiting following BEAM chemotherapy before autologous hematopoietic stem cell transplantation. Transplant Proc 43(8):3107–3110
48. Badar T, Cortes J, Borthakur G, O'Brien S, Wierda W, Garcia-Manero G, Ferrajoli A, Kadia T, Poku R, Kantarjian H, Mattiuzzi G (2015) Phase II, open label, randomized comparative trial of ondansetron alone versus the combination of ondansetron and aprepitant for the prevention of nausea and vomiting in patients with hematologic malignancies receiving regimens containing high-dose cytarabine. Biomed Res Int 2015:497597
49. Egerer G, Eisenlohr K, Gronkowski M, Burhenne J, Riedel KD, Mikus G (2010) The NK(1) receptor antagonist aprepitant does not alter the pharmacokinetics of high-dose melphalan chemotherapy in patients with multiple myeloma. Br J Clin Pharmacol 70(6):903–907
50. Schmitt T, Goldschmidt H, Neben K, Freiberger A, Hüsing J, Gronkowski M, Thalheimer M, le Pelzl H, Mikus G, Burhenne J, Ho AD, Egerer G (2014) Aprepitant, granisetron, and dexamethasone for prevention of chemotherapy-induced nausea and vomiting after high-dose melphalan in autologous transplantation for multiple myeloma: results of a randomized, placebo-controlled phase III trial. J Clin Oncol 32(30):3413–3420
51. Bechtel T, McBride A, Crawford B, Bullington S, Hofmeister CC, Benson DM Jr, Jaglowski S, Penza S, Andritsos LA, Devine SM (2014) Aprepitant for the control of delayed nausea and vomiting associated with the use of high-dose melphalan for autologous peripheral blood stem cell transplants in patients with multiple myeloma: a phase II study. Support Care Cancer 22(11):2911–2916
52. dos Santos LV, Souza FH, Brunetto AT, Sasse AD, da Silveira Nogueira Lima JP (2012) Neurokinin-1 receptor antagonists for chemotherapy-induced nausea and vomiting: a systematic review. J Natl Cancer Inst 104(17):1280–1292
53. Chawla SP, Grunberg SM, Gralla RJ, Hesketh PJ, Rittenberg C, Elmer ME, Schmidt C, Taylor A, Carides AD, Evans JK, Horgan KJ (2003) Establishing the dose of the oral NK1 antagonist aprepitant for the prevention of chemotherapy-induced nausea and vomiting. Cancer 97(9):2290–2300
54. Leal AD, Kadakia KC, Looker S, Hilger C, Sorgatz K, Anderson K, Jacobson A, Grendahl D, Seisler D, Hobday T, Loprinzi CL (2014) Fosaprepitant-induced phlebitis: a focus on patients receiving doxorubicin/cyclophosphamide therapy. Support Care Cancer 22(5):1313–1317
55. Aapro MS, Walko CM (2010) Aprepitant: drug-drug interactions in perspective. Ann Oncol 21(12):2316–2323

56. Shadle CR, Lee Y, Majumdar AK, Petty KJ, Gargano C, Bradstreet TE, Evans JK, Blum RA (2004) Evaluation of potential inductive effects of aprepitant on cytochrome P450 3A4 and 2C9 activity. J Clin Pharmacol 44(3):215–223
57. de Jonge ME, Huitema AD, Holtkamp MJ, van Dam SM, Beijnen JH, Rodenhuis S (2005) Aprepitant inhibits cyclophosphamide bioactivation and thiotepa metabolism. Cancer Chemother Pharmacol 56(4):370–378
58. Rapoport BL, Weinstein C, Camacho ES, Khanani SA, Beckford-Brathwaite E, Kevill L, Vallejos W, Liang LW, Noga SJ (2015) A phase III, randomized, double-blind study of single-dose intravenous fosaprepitant in preventing chemotherapy-induced nausea and vomiting associated with moderately emetogenic chemotherapy. J Clin Oncol 33(Suppl; abstr 9629)
59. Albany C, Brames MJ, Fausel C, Johnson CS, Picus J, Einhorn LH (2012) Randomized, double-blind, placebo-controlled, phase III cross-over study evaluating the oral neurokinin-1 antagonist aprepitant in combination with a 5HT3 receptor antagonist and dexamethasone in patients with germ cell tumors receiving 5-day cisplatin combination chemotherapy regimens: a hoosier oncology group study. J Clin Oncol 30(32):3998–4003

Chapter 6
Olanzapine for the Prevention of Chemotherapy-Induced Nausea and Vomiting

Rudolph M. Navari

6.1 Introduction

6.1.1 Chemotherapy-Induced Nausea and Vomiting

Chemotherapy-induced nausea and vomiting (CINV) is associated with a significant deterioration in quality of life and is perceived by patients as a major adverse effect of the treatment [1]. The use of 5-hydroxytryptamine-3 (5-HT$_3$) receptor antagonists plus dexamethasone has significantly improved the control of CINV [2]. Recent studies have demonstrated additional improvement in the control of CINV with the use of new agents: palonosetron, a second generation 5-HT$_3$ receptor antagonist [3]; NK-1 receptor antagonists aprepitant, netupitant, and rolapitant [4–6]; and olanzapine, an antipsychotic which blocks multiple neurotransmitters in the central nervous system [7–9].

The primary end point used for studies evaluating various agents for the control of CINV has been complete response (CR) (no emesis, no use of rescue medication) over the acute (24 h post-chemotherapy), delayed (24–120 h), and overall (0–120 h) periods [2]. Recent studies have shown that the combination of a 5-HT$_3$ receptor antagonist, dexamethasone, and a NK1 receptor antagonist have been very effective in controlling emesis in patients receiving either highly emetogenic chemotherapy (HEC) or moderately emetogenic chemotherapy (MEC) over a 120 h period following chemotherapy administration [4–6]. Many of these same studies have measured

R.M. Navari, MD, PhD, FACP
Cancer Care Program, Central and South America, World Health Organization,
Atlanta, USA

Student Outreach Clinic, Indiana University School of Medicine South Bend,
South Bend, IN, USA
e-mail: rmnavari@gmail.com

© Springer International Publishing Switzerland 2016
R.M. Navari (ed.), *Management of Chemotherapy-Induced Nausea
and Vomiting: New Agents and New Uses of Current Agents*,
DOI 10.1007/978-3-319-27016-6_6

nausea as a secondary end point and have demonstrated that nausea has not been well controlled [10].

Emesis is a well-defined event which is easily measured, but nausea may be more subjective and more difficult to measure. There are, however, two well-defined measures of nausea which appear to be effective measurement tools which are reproducible: the visual analogue scale (VAS) and the Likert scale [11]. The VAS is a scale from 0 to 10 or 0 to 100 with zero representing no nausea and 10 or 100 representing maximal nausea. The Likert scale asks patients to rate nausea as none, mild, moderate, or severe.

6.1.2 Definition of Nausea

Nausea is a subjective, difficult to describe, sick, or queasy sensation, usually perceived as being in the stomach that is sometimes followed by emesis [11]. The experience of nausea is difficult to describe in another person because it is a subjective sensation. Nausea and emesis are not necessarily on a continuum. One can experience nausea without emesis and one can have sudden emesis without nausea. Nausea has been assumed to be the conscious awareness of unusual sensations in the "vomiting center" of the brainstem (Fig. 6.1), but the existence of such a center and its relationship to nausea remain controversial [11].

Figure 6.2 illustrates the various receptors that are considered to be involved in CINV.

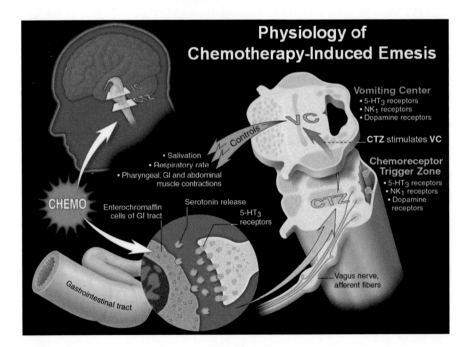

Fig. 6.1 Physiology of chemotherapy-induced emesis

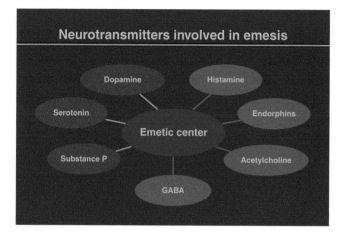

Fig. 6.2 Neurotransmitters involved in emesis

These receptors are located both in the periphery such as the gastrointestinal tract and in the central nervous system. Various antiemetic agents have been developed as antagonists to the serotonin and the substance P receptors with relative success in controlling emesis. It is not clear whether the serotonin and/or the substance P receptors are important in the control of nausea.

Other receptors such as dopaminergic, histaminic, and muscarinic may be the dominant receptors in the control of nausea [8, 10].

6.2   Olanzapine

6.2.1   Mechanism of Action

Olanzapine, an atypical antipsychotic agent of the thienobenzodiazepine class, was approved by the FDA for the treatment of the manifestations of psychotic disorders in 1996 [12, 13] with a generic available in 2011. Olanzapine blocks multiple neurotransmitter receptors including dopaminergic at D_1, D_2, D_3, and D_4 brain receptors; serotonergic at 5-HT_{2a}, 5-HT_{2c}, 5-HT_3, and 5-HT_6 receptors; catecholamines at alpha_1 adrenergic receptors; acetylcholine at muscarinic receptors; and histamine at H_1 receptors [14]. Olanzapine has five times the affinity for 5-HT_2 receptors than D_2 receptors [15] and is used to treat schizophrenia and delirium [16, 17]. Olanzapine may reduce opioid requirements in cancer patients with uncontrolled pain, cognitive impairment, or anxiety [18].

The detailed mechanism of the effect of olanzapine in reducing CINV is unknown, but olanzapine does block the neurotransmitters dopamine and serotonin which are known mediators of CINV [14, 19]. Olanzapine blocks the serotonin-mediated 5-HT_{2C} receptor, a receptor which has been shown to mediate antiemetic activity in animal models (ferret cisplatin-induced emesis and cisplatin-induced anorexia in the hypothalamus of rats) [20, 21] as well as weight loss in humans [22].

The effect of olanzapine on this receptor as well as other dopamine and serotonin receptors may explain in part its efficacy in CINV.

A benefit of olanzapine is that it is not a cytochrome P450 inhibitor and appears to have few drug interactions [14].

Common side effects are sedation and weight gain [23, 24], as well as an association with the onset of diabetes mellitus [25].

6.2.2 Treatment of Nausea/Case Reports

There have been case reports on the use of olanzapine as an antinausea agent [26–31]. A patient with leukemia reported a significant improvement in chronic nausea with the use of olanzapine [30], and in six patients receiving palliative care, olanzapine was found to be effective for intractable nausea due to opioids, neoplasm, and/or medications [26]. Olanzapine was effective in controlling refractory nausea and vomiting in two patients with advanced cancer [31]. In a case report, olanzapine was effective in controlling opioid-induced nausea [32], and in an open label trial, olanzapine was effective in reducing nausea in 15 advanced cancer patients with opioid-induced nausea [29]. In a retrospective chart review of 28 patients who received olanzapine on a needed basis following moderate to highly emetogenic chemotherapy, the data suggested that olanzapine may decrease delayed emesis [28].

Bowel obstruction is one of the most common complications in patients with advanced cancer either due to the ingestion of pain medications, large or small intestinal dysfunction, or other tumor-induced issues [13]. A retrospective study carried out on a palliative care unit demonstrated that in 18 of 20 patients, the use of olanzapine led to a significant decrease in the average intensity score of nausea, suggesting a role for olanzapine in the relief of nausea in patients with incomplete bowel obstruction [13].

Based on the above, it appears that olanzapine has significant potential for use in the prevention and treatment of nausea in a palliative care setting as well as patients with opioid-induced nausea. Due to its mechanism of action of blocking multiple neurotransmitter receptors, it can be used as a single agent, and due to its long half-life, it can be given as once-daily dosing that would improve patient compliance.

6.2.3 Prevention of Chemotherapy-Induced Nausea and Vomiting

6.2.3.1 Phase I Trial

The case reports discussed above prompted a phase I study in which olanzapine was added to the prophylactic antiemetics granisetron and dexamethasone in cancer patients receiving their first cycle of chemotherapy in order to determine the maximum tolerated dose as an antiemetic [33]. The phase I study was designed with olanzapine, utilizing a four-cohort dose escalation of three to six patients per cohort, for the prevention of delayed emesis in cancer patients receiving chemotherapy consisting of cyclophosphamide, doxorubicin, platinum, and/or irinotecan. Olanzapine was administered on days 2 and 1 prior to chemotherapy and continued for 8 days (days 0–7). Episodes of vomiting as well as daily measurements of nausea, sedation, and toxicity were monitored at each dose level. Fifteen patients completed the protocol. No Grade 4 toxicities were seen, and three patients experienced a dose-limiting toxicity (Grade 3) of a depressed level of consciousness during the study. The maximum tolerated dose appeared to be 5 mg (for days 2 and 1) and 10 mg (for days 0–7). Four of six patients receiving HEC (cisplatin, ≥ 70 mg/m^2) and nine of nine patients receiving MEC (doxorubicin, ≥ 50 mg/m^2) had a CR of delayed emesis. Using the maximum tolerated dose of olanzapine in the phase I trial, a phase II trial was performed for the prevention of chemotherapy-induced nausea and vomiting in patients receiving their first course of either HEC or MEC.

6.2.3.2   Phase II Trials

Using the maximum tolerated dose of olanzapine in the previously described phase I trial [33], a phase II trial was performed for the prevention of chemotherapy-induced nausea and vomiting in chemotherapy-naive patients. The regimen was 5 mg/day of oral olanzapine on the 2 days prior to chemotherapy; 10 mg of olanzapine on the day of chemotherapy, day 1 (added to intravenous granisetron, 10 mcg/kg and dexamethasone, 20 mg); and 10 mg/day on days 2–4 after chemotherapy (added to dexamethasone, 8 mg p.o. BID, days 2, 3 and 4 mg p.o. BID, day 4). Thirty patients (median age 58.5 years, range 25–84; 23 females; ECOG PS 0,1) consented to the protocol and all were evaluable. CR was 100 % for the acute period (24 h post-chemotherapy), 80 % for the delayed period (days 2–5 post-chemotherapy), and 80 % for the overall period (0–120 h post-chemotherapy) in ten patients receiving HEC (cisplatin, ≥ 70 mg/m^2). CR was also 100 % for the acute period, 85 % for the delayed period, and 85 % for the overall period in 20 patients receiving MEC (doxorubicin, ≥ 50 mg/m^2). Nausea was very well controlled in the patients receiving HEC with no patient having nausea (0 on a scale of 0–10, MD Anderson Symptom Inventory (MDASI)) in the acute or delayed periods. Nausea was also well controlled in patients receiving MEC with no nausea in 85 % of patients in the acute period and 65 % in the delayed and overall periods. There were no Grade 3 or 4 toxicities and no significant pain, fatigue, disturbed sleep, memory changes, dyspnea, lack of appetite, drowsiness, dry mouth, mood changes, or restlessness experienced by the patients. CR and control of nausea in subsequent cycles of chemotherapy (25 patients, cycle 2; 25 patients, cycle 3; 21 patients, cycle 4) were equal to or greater than cycle 1. Based on this phase II study, olanzapine appeared to be safe and highly effective in controlling acute and delayed chemotherapy-induced nausea and vomiting in patients receiving HEC and MEC [34].

An additional phase II study was performed with olanzapine to determine the control of acute and delayed chemotherapy-induced nausea and vomiting (CINV) in patients receiving MEC and HEC with the combined use of palonosetron, olanzapine, and dexamethasone with the dexamethasone given on day 1 only. Forty chemotherapy-naïve patients received on the day of chemotherapy, day 1, an antiemetic regimen consisting of dexamethasone, palonosetron, and olanzapine. Patients continued olanzapine for days 2–4 following chemotherapy administration. Patients recorded daily episodes of emesis, daily symptoms utilizing the MD Anderson Symptom Inventory, and the utilization of rescue therapy. For the first cycle of chemotherapy, the CR for the acute period (24 h post-chemotherapy) was 100 %, the delayed period (days 2–5 post-chemotherapy) 75 %, and the overall period (0–120 h post-chemotherapy) 75 % in 8 patients receiving HEC and was 97 %, 75 %, and 72 % in 32 patients receiving MEC. Patients with no nausea for the acute period was 100 %, the delayed period 50 %, and the overall period 50 % in 8 patients receiving HEC and was 100 %, 78 %, and 78 % in 32 patients receiving MEC. The CR and control of nausea in subsequent cycles of chemotherapy were not significantly different from cycle 1. Olanzapine combined with a single dose of dexamethasone and a single dose of palonosetron was very effective in controlling acute and delayed CINV in patients receiving both HEC and MEC [35].

Compared to the previous phase I and phase II studies, olanzapine was given for only 4 days (the day of chemotherapy and 3 days post-chemotherapy), and there was no dexamethasone given post-chemotherapy in the delayed period. Despite the reduced number of daily doses of olanzapine and dexamethasone, the antiemetic regimen was highly effective in the prevention of chemotherapy-induced nausea and vomiting in patients receiving MEC or HEC.

6.2.3.3   Phase III Trials

A phase III study was designed to evaluate the activity and safety of olanzapine compared with 5-HT$_3$ receptor antagonists for the prevention of chemotherapy-induced nausea and vomiting in patients receiving HEC or MEC [9]. The study also evaluated the impact of olanzapine on the quality of life of cancer patients during the chemotherapy period.

Two hundred twenty-nine patients receiving MEC or HEC were randomly assigned to azasetron (day 1), dexamethasone (day 1), and olanzapine (days 1–5) or to azasetron (day 1) and dexamethasone (days 1–5). The primary end point was CR for the acute period (24 h post-chemotherapy), delayed period (24–120 h post-chemotherapy), and overall period (0–120 h post-chemotherapy). The secondary end points were quality of life post-chemotherapy, safety, and toxicity. CR was significantly improved for patients receiving either MEC or HEC for the olanzapine group in the delayed and the overall periods (Figs. 6.3 and 6.4). There was no difference between the groups for the acute period. The patients receiving olanzapine had a significant improvement in global health status, emotional functioning, social functioning, fatigue, insomnia, and appetite loss. Seventy-three percent of the patients who received olanzapine reported sleepiness during the chemo-

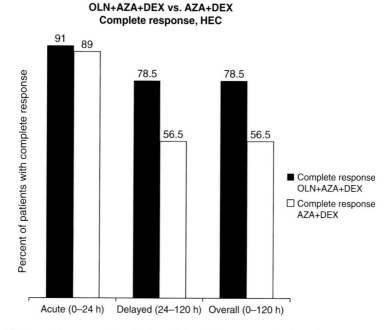

Fig. 6.3 Complete response in patients receiving highly emetogenic chemotherapy

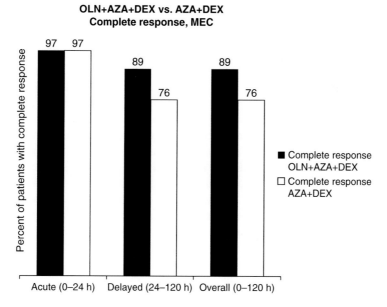

Fig. 6.4 Complete response in patients receiving moderately emetogenic chemotherapy

therapy, but there were no Grade 3 or 4 toxicities. The side effect of sleepiness may have effectively relieved insomnia and agitation which can be caused by dexamethasone. The study concluded that olanzapine improved the CR of delayed CINV and quality of life in patients receiving MEC and HEC. Olanzapine was safe with no Grade 3 or 4 toxicities [9].

An additional phase III study was recently performed to compare the effectiveness of olanzapine and aprepitant for the prevention of chemotherapy-induced nausea and vomiting in patients receiving HEC [7]. Chemotherapy-naïve patients receiving cisplatin ($\geq$70 mg/m^2) or cyclophosphamide ($\geq$500 mg/m^2) and doxorubicin ($\geq$50 mg/m^2) were randomized to either olanzapine or aprepitant in combination with palonosetron and dexamethasone. The olanzapine regimen was 10 mg of oral olanzapine, 0.25 mg of IV palonosetron, 20 mg IV pre-chemotherapy of dexamethasone on day 1 and 10 mg/day of oral olanzapine alone on days 2–4 post-chemotherapy. The aprepitant, palonosetron, and dexamethasone regimen was 125 mg of oral aprepitant, 0.25 mg IV palonosetron, and 12 mg IV of dexamethasone on day 1 and 80 mg oral aprepitant with 4 mg dexamethasone BID on days 2 and 3. Two hundred and fifty-one patients consented to the protocol and were randomized. Two hundred forty-one patients were evaluable. CR was 97 % for the acute period (24 h post-chemotherapy), 77 % for the delayed period (days 2–5 post-chemotherapy), and 77 % for the overall period (0–120 h) for 121 patients receiving the olanzapine regimen. CR was 87 % for the acute period, 73 % for the delayed period, and 73 % for the overall period in 120 patients receiving the aprepitant regimen. Patients without nausea (0, scale 0–10, M.D. Anderson Symptom Inventory) were placed on olanzapine regimen at 87%, acute; 69%, delayed; and 69%, overall and aprepitant regimen at 87%, acute; 38%, delayed; and 38%, overall (Fig. 6.5). There were no Grade 3 or 4 toxicities. Grade I or II levels of sedation were not available from the study. CR and control of nausea in subsequent chemotherapy cycles were equal to or greater than cycle 1 for both regimens. Olanzapine, palonosetron, and dexamethasone were comparable to aprepitant, palonosetron, and dexamethasone in the control of chemotherapy-induced emesis. Nausea was significantly better controlled with olanzapine, palonosetron, and dexamethasone [7].

The benefit of olanzapine for decreasing nausea has been demonstrated in another trial. In a randomized, double-blind, placebo-controlled design [36], 44 patients scheduled to receive MEC or HEC received a 5-HT$_3$ receptor antagonist, dexamethasone, and a NK-1 receptor antagonist. Patients were then randomized to receive 5 mg of olanzapine daily or placebo for 6 days beginning on the day before chemotherapy or placebo. CR rates and freedom from nausea were significantly improved in the patients receiving olanzapine.

A recently completed randomized, double-blind, phase III trial was performed using olanzapine for the prevention of CINV in chemotherapy-naïve patients receiving cisplatin, $\geq$70 mg/m^2 or cyclophosphamide-anthracycline-based chemotherapy, comparing OLN to placebo in combination with aprepitant, a 5-HT$_3$ receptor antagonist, and dexamethasone. In this trial, complete freedom from nausea was the primary end point, and complete response was a secondary end point. The olanzapine regimen was significantly more effective for the control of nausea and numerically had a higher complete response rate in the acute, delayed, and overall periods [37].

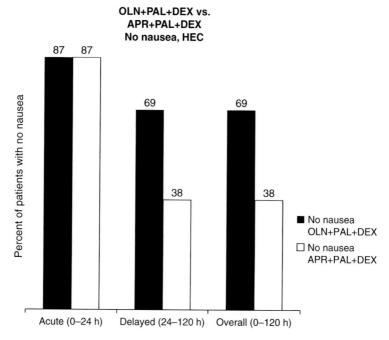

Fig. 6.5   No nausea in patients receiving highly emetogenic chemotherapy

6.3   Treatment of Breakthrough Chemotherapy-Induced Nausea and Vomiting

Despite the improved control of acute and delayed CINV with new agents, breakthrough CINV, nausea, and emesis which occurs despite adequate antiemetic prophylaxis remains a significant patient problem [38]. No randomized, double-blind trials have investigated the use of antiemetics in the treatment of breakthrough CINV [39]. The Multinational Association of Supportive Care in Cancer (MASCC) [39] and the American Society of Clinical Oncology (ASCO) [40] guidelines have suggested that when breakthrough CINV occurs, the prophylactic regimen in subsequent chemotherapy cycles should be changed by switching to a different 5-HT$_3$ receptor antagonist, substituting metoclopramide for the 5-HT$_3$ receptor antagonist, or adding other agents such as dopamine antagonists or benzodiazepines [39, 40]. These guidelines do not suggest a treatment for breakthrough CINV. The National Comprehensive Cancer Network (NCCN) (www.nccn.org) guidelines suggest treating breakthrough CINV with an agent from a drug class that was not used in the prophylactic regimen and recommend continuing the breakthrough medication if nausea and vomiting is controlled.

Agents used for the prevention of nausea and vomiting have not been studied for the treatment of established nausea and vomiting [41], and the National Cancer Institute's Physician Data Query (PDQ) for supportive care states that there is no known effective therapy for treatment of nausea and vomiting that occurs after chemotherapy (www.cancer.gov/cancertopics/pdq.supportivecare/nausea/healthprofessional).

In a recent study, olanzapine was compared to metoclopramide for the treatment of breakthrough CINV in chemotherapy-naïve patients receiving HEC and guideline-directed prophylactic antiemetics [8]. Both metoclopramide and olanzapine have been recommended as single agents for the treatment of breakthrough CINV (NCCN), but no study has reported the effectiveness of either of these agents for breakthrough CINV.

Metoclopramide is a dopamine receptor antagonist which acts at dopamine receptors in the gastrointestinal tract and in the chemoreceptor zone located in the area postrema [8].

Prior to the development of the serotonin receptor antagonists, dopamine receptor antagonists were used extensively for the prevention of CINV. Metoclopramide is FDA approved for the treatment of nausea and vomiting, as well as the prevention of CINV and the prevention of postoperative nausea and vomiting [8].

Since olanzapine has been shown to be a safe and effective agent for the prevention of CINV, olanzapine may also be an effective rescue medication for patients who develop breakthrough CINV despite having received guideline-directed CINV prophylaxis. A double-blind, randomized phase III trial was performed for the treatment of breakthrough CINV in chemotherapy-naïve patients receiving HEC (cisplatin, ≥ 70 mg/m^2 or doxorubicin, ≥ 50 mg/m^2 and cyclophosphamide, ≥ 600 mg/m^2) comparing olanzapine to metoclopramide. Patients who developed breakthrough emesis or nausea despite prophylactic dexamethasone (12 mg IV), palonosetron (0.25 mg IV), and fosaprepitant (150 mg IV) pre-chemotherapy and dexamethasone (8 mg p.o. daily, days 2–4) post-chemotherapy were randomized to receive olanzapine 10 mg orally daily for 3 days or metoclopramide 10 mg orally TID for 3 days. Patients were monitored for emesis and nausea for the 72 h after taking olanzapine or metoclopramide.

Two hundred seventy-six patients (median age 56 years, range 38–79; 43 females; ECOG PS 0, 1) consented to the protocol. One hundred twelve patients developed breakthrough CINV and 108 were evaluable. During the 72 h observation period, 39 of 56 (70 %) patients receiving olanzapine had no emesis compared to 16 of 52 (31 %) patients with no emesis receiving metoclopramide ($p<0.01$). Patients without nausea (0, scale 0–10, MD Anderson Symptom Inventory) during the 72 h observation period were olanzapine 68 % (38 of 56) and metoclopramide 23 % (12 of 52) ($p<0.01$). There was no Grade 3 or 4 toxicities. In this study, olanzapine was significantly better than metoclopramide in the control of breakthrough emesis and nausea in patients receiving HEC. This was the first randomized phase III clinical trial on the treatment of breakthrough emesis and nausea [8].

6.4 Future Applications

Although there have been significant improvements in the prevention of chemotherapy-induced nausea and vomiting in patients receiving single-day HEC and MEC, there has been limited progress in the prevention of chemotherapy-induced nausea and vomiting in patients receiving multiple-day chemotherapy or high-dose chemotherapy with stem cell transplant. The current recommendation is to give a first-generation 5-HT$_3$ receptor antagonist and dexamethasone daily during each day of chemotherapy in patients receiving multiple-day chemotherapy or high-dose chemotherapy with stem cell transplant [42]. This regimen appears to be at least partially effective in controlling acute chemotherapy-induced nausea and vomiting but is not very effective in controlling delayed chemotherapy-induced nausea and vomiting. The CR in most studies of 5 days of cisplatin and in various high-dose chemotherapy regimens is 30–70 %, with the majority of studies reporting a CR of ≤50 % [42].

Patients should receive the appropriate prophylaxis for the emetogenic risk of the chemotherapy for each day of the chemotherapy treatment. Both acute and delayed chemotherapy-induced nausea and vomiting may occur on day 2 or subsequent chemotherapy days and delayed chemotherapy-induced nausea and vomiting may occur after the last day of the multi-day chemotherapy treatment.

Olanzapine has been shown to be effective in controlling both acute and delayed chemotherapy-induced nausea and vomiting in patients receiving single-day MEC and HEC. Olanzapine may have application in patients receiving multiple-day or high-dose chemotherapy. Palonosetron has been used in one report of patients receiving 5 days of cisplatin [43], and Albany et al. [44] reported that the addition of aprepitant to a 5-HT$_3$ receptor antagonist and dexamethasone significantly improved the CR in patients receiving 5 days of cisplatin.

Olanzapine has not been studied extensively in multi-day chemotherapy, bone marrow transplantation, or radiotherapy-induced nausea and vomiting. Future studies may address whether olanzapine would be effective in patients who experience nausea and vomiting during these clinical settings. Future studies may determine not only how olanzapine may be used and what combinations of new and older agents will be the most beneficial for patients but may also provide new information on the mechanism of chemotherapy-induced nausea and vomiting.

6.5   Conclusions

Olanzapine is an atypical antipsychotic agent of the thienobenzodiazepine class that blocks multiple neurotransmitter receptors including the D$_2$, 5-HT$_{2c}$, and 5-HT$_3$ receptors which appear to be involved in nausea and emesis. It has a potential role in the treatment of nausea and vomiting refractory to standard antiemetics. Clinical reports suggest that it is effective in the treatment of chronic nausea in patients receiving palliative care and for patients with intractable nausea due to opioids, neoplasm, and/or medications. Phase II and phase III clinical trials have demonstrated its effectiveness in the prevention of chemotherapy-induced acute and delayed nausea and vomiting with significant more effectiveness in preventing nausea than current antiemetics used in the prophylaxis of chemotherapy-induced nausea and vomiting. A recent trial also demonstrated effectiveness in treating breakthrough chemotherapy-induced nausea and vomiting.

The benefit of olanzapine for decreasing nausea is in contrast to the control of nausea in clinical trials of the NK-1 receptor antagonists. Nausea has not been significantly improved by the use of aprepitant [4], netupitant [5], or rolapitant [6]. Two reviews on the prevention of chemotherapy-induced nausea concluded that NK-1 receptor antagonists are not effective in controlling nausea [4, 10].

The data from the olanzapine clinical trials discussed above support NCCN guidelines which list the olanzapine, palonosetron, and dexamethasone regimen as an optional first-line therapy for the prevention of CINV in patients receiving HEC and MEC [45].

There are economic benefits of olanzapine. Four days of generic oral olanzapine at 10 mg/day, the dose used in previous prophylactic studies [8, 9, 34, 35, 37], is approximately $3.00 [46] which is significantly lower than the cost of 1 day of intravenous fosaprepitant at 150 mg (approximate wholesale acquisition cost: $257.00) [47].

Olanzapine appears to be well tolerated in the reported clinical trials. The recently completed phase III clinical trial involving a large number of patients receiving olanzapine reported no significant toxicities in patients receiving 4 days of olanzapine [37]. Patients who received olanzapine had more drowsiness on day 2 post-chemotherapy compared to baseline, but this resolved by day 3 despite continued oral olanzapine on days 3 and 4, suggesting that patients adapted to the olanzapine. Due to the temporary drowsiness seen in this trial and reports of temporary drowsiness in some patients, more detailed data on drowsiness ratings should be obtained in future trials.

Olanzapine has not been studied extensively in multi-day chemotherapy, bone marrow transplantation, or radiotherapy-induced nausea and vomiting. Future studies may address whether olanzapine would be effective in patients who experience nausea and vomiting during these clinical settings.

References

1. Bloechl-Daum B, Deuson RR, Mavros P, Hansen M, Herrstedt J (2006) Delayed nausea and vomiting continue to reduce patients' quality of life after highly and moderately emetogenic chemotherapy despite antiemetic treatment. J Clin Oncol 24:4472–4478
2. Navari RM (2013) Management of chemotherapy-induced nausea and vomiting: focus on newer agents and new uses for older agents. Drugs 73:249–262
3. Navari RM (2013) The current status of the use of palonosetron. Expert Opin Pharmacother 14:1281–1284
4. Aapro M, Carides A, Rapoport BL (2015) Aprepitant and fosaprepitant: a ten-year review of efficacy and safety. Oncologist 20:450–458
5. Navari RM (2015) Profile of netupitant/palonosetron fixed dose combination (NEPA) and its potential in the treatment of chemotherapy-induced nausea and vomiting (CINV). Drug Des Dev Ther 9:155–161
6. Navari RM (2015) Rolapitant for the treatment of chemotherapy induced nausea and vomiting. Expert Rev Anticancer Ther 15:1127–1133
7. Navari RM, Gray SE, Kerr AC (2011) Olanzapine versus aprepitant for the prevention of chemotherapy-induced nausea and vomiting: a randomized phase III trial. J Support Oncol 9:188–195

8. Navari RM, Nagy CK, Gray SE (2013) Olanzapine versus metoclopramide for the treatment of breakthrough chemotherapy-induced nausea and vomiting in patients receiving highly emetogenic chemotherapy. Support Care Cancer 21:1655–1663
9. Tan L, Liu J, Liu X, Chen J, Yan Z, Yang H, Zhang D (2009) Clinical research of olanzapine for the prevention of chemotherapy-induced nausea and vomiting. J Exp Clin Cancer Res 28:1–7
10. Navari RM (2012) Treatment of chemotherapy-induced nausea. Community Oncol 9:20–26
11. Stern RM, Koch KL, Andrews PLR (2011) Nausea: mechanisms and management. Oxford University Press, Oxford/New York
12. Fulton B, Goa KL (1997) Olanzapine: a review of its pharmacological properties and therapeutic efficacy in the management of schizophrenia and related psychoses. Drugs 53:281–298
13. Kando JC, Shepski JC, Satterlee W, Patel JK, Rearns SG, Green AL (1997) Olanzapine: a new antipsychotic agent with efficacy in the management of schizophrenia. Ann Pharmacother 31:1325–1334
14. Bymaster FP, Calligaro D, Falcone J, Marsh RD, Moore NA, Tye NC, Seeman P, Wong DT (1996) Radioreceptor binding profile of the atypical antipsychotic olanzapine. Neuropsychopharmacology 14:87–96
15. Stephenson CME, Pilowsky LS (1999) Psychopharmacology of olanzapine: a review. Br J Psychiatry 174:52–58
16. Breithart W, Tremblay A, Gibson C (2002) An open trial of olanzapine for the treatment of delirium in hospitalized cancer patients. Psychosomatics 43:175–182
17. Kim KS, Pae CU, Chae JH, Bahk WM, Jun T (2001) An open pilot trial of olanzapine for delirium for the Korean population. Psychiatry Clin Neurosci 55:515–519
18. Khojainova N, Santiago-Palma J, Kornick C, Breitbart W, Gonzales GR (2002) Olanzapine in the management of cancer pain. J Pain Symptom Manage 23:546–550
19. Bymaster FP, Falcone JF, Bauzon D, Kennedy JS, Schenck K, DeLapp NW, Cohen ML (2001) Potent antagonism of 5-HT(3) and 5-HT(6) receptors by olanzapine. Eur J Pharmacol 430:341–349
20. Rudd JA, Ngan MP, Wai MK, King AG, Witherington J, Andrews PL, Sanger GJ (2006) Antiemetic activity of ghrelin in ferrets exposed to the cytotoxic anti-cancer agent cisplatin. Neurosci Lett 392:79–83
21. Yakabi K, Sadakane C, Noguchi M, Ohno S, Shoki R, Chinen K, Aoyanna T, Sakurada T, Takabayashi H, Hattori T (2010) Reduced ghrelin secretion in the hypothalamus of rats due to cisplatin-induced anorexia. Endocrinology 151:3773–3782
22. Hurren KM, Berlie HD (2011) Lorcaserin: an investigational serotonin 2C agonist for weight loss. Am J Health Syst Pharm 68:2029–2037
23. Allison DB, Casey DE (2001) Antipsychotic-associated weight gain: a review of the literature. J Clin Psychiatry 62:22–31
24. Hale AS (1997) Olanzapine. Br J Hosp Med 58:443–445
25. Goldstein LE, Sporn J, Brown S, Kim H, Finkelstein J, Gaffey GK, Sachs G, Stern TA (1999) New-onset diabetes mellitus and diabetic ketoacidosis associated with olanzapine treatment. Psychosomatics 40:438–443
26. Jackson WC, Tavernier L (2003) Olanzapine for intractable nausea in palliative care patients. J Palliat Med 6:251–255
27. Licup N, Baumrucker S (2010) Olanzapine for nausea and vomiting. Am J Hosp Palliat Care 27:432–434
28. Passik SD, Kirsh KL, Theobald DE, Dickerson P, Trowbridge R, Gray D, Beaver M, Comparet J, Brown J (2003) A retrospective chart review of the use of olanzapine for the prevention of delayed emesis in cancer patients. J Pain Symptom Manage 25:485–489
29. Passik SD, Lundberg J, Kirsh KL, Theobald D, Donagby K, Holtschaw E, Cooper M, Dugan W (2002) Clinical note: a pilot exploration of the antiemetic activity of olanzapine for the relief of nausea in patients with advanced pain and cancer. J Pain Symptom Manage 23:526–532
30. Pirl WF, Roth AJ (2000) Remission of chemotherapy-induced emesis with concurrent olanzapine treatment: a case report. Psychooncology 9:84–87

31. Srivastava M, Brito-Dellan N, Davis MP, Leach M, Lagman R (2003) Olanzapine as an anti-
    emetic in refractory nausea and vomiting in advanced cancer. J Pain Symptom Manage
    25:578–582
32. Lundberg JC, Passik S (2000) Controlling opioid-induced nausea with olanzapine. Prim Care
    Cancer 20:35–37
33. Passik S, Navari RM, Jung SH, Nagy CK, Vinson J, Kirsh KL, Loehrer PJ (2004) A phase I
    trial of olanzapine for the prevention of delayed emesis in cancer patients receiving chemo-
    therapy. Cancer Invest 22:383–388
34. Navari RM, Einhorn LH, Passik SD, Loehrer PJ, Johnson C, Mayer ML, McClean J, Vinson J,
    Pletcher W (2005) A phase II trial of olanzapine for the prevention of chemotherapy-induced
    nausea and vomiting. Support Care Cancer 13:529–534
35. Navari RM, Einhorn LH, Loehrer PJ, Passik SD, Vinson J, McClean J, Chowhan N, Hanna
    NH, Johnson CS (2007) A phase II trial of olanzapine, dexamethasone, and palonosetron for
    the prevention of chemotherapy-induced nausea and vomiting. Support Care Cancer
    15:1285–1291
36. Mizukami N, Yamanchi M, Koike K et al (2014) Olanzapine for the prevention of
    chemotherapy-induced nausea and vomiting in patients receiving highly or moderately emeto-
    genic chemotherapy: a randomized, double-blind, placebo-controlled study. J Pain Symptom
    Manage 47:542–550
37. Navari RM, Qin R, Ruddy KJ et al (2015) Olanzapine for the prevention of chemotherapy-
    induced nausea and vomiting (CINV) in patients receiving highly emetogenic chemotherapy
    (HEC): alliance: A221301, a randomized, double-blind, placebo-controlled trial. ASCO pal-
    liative care symposium, abstract 176, Boston
38. Tina Shih YC, Xu Y, Elting LS (2007) Costs of uncontrolled chemotherapy-induced nausea
    and vomiting among working-age cancer patients receiving highly or moderately emetogenic
    chemotherapy. Cancer 110:678–685
39. Roila F, Herrstedt J, Aapro M, Gralla RJ, Einhorn LH, Ballatori E, Bria E, Clark-Snow RA,
    Espersen BT, Feyer P, Grunberg SM, Hesketh PJ, Jordan K, Kris MG, Maranzano A, Morrow
    G, Oliver I, Rapoport BL, Rittenberg C, Saito M, Tonato M, Warr D (2010) Guideline update
    for MASCC and ESMO in the prevention of chemotherapy- and radiotherapy-induced nausea
    and vomiting: results of the Perugia consensus conference. Ann Oncol 21:232–243
40. Basch E, Prestrud AA, Hesketh PJ, Kris MG, Fever PC, Somerfield MR, Chesney M, Clark-
    Snow RA, Flaherty AM, Freunlich B, Morrow G, Rao KV, Schwartz RN, Lyman GH (2011)
    Antiemetic American Society Clinical Oncology clinical practice guideline update. J Clin
    Oncol 29:4189–4198
41. Kris MC (2003) Why do we need another antiemetic? Just ask. J Clin Oncol 21:4077–4080
42. Navari RM (2007) Prevention of emesis from multiple-day chemotherapy regimens. J Natl
    Compr Canc Netw 5:51–59
43. Einhorn LH, Brames ML, Dreicer R, Nichols CR, Cullen MT, Bubalo J (2007) Palonosetron
    plus dexamethasone for the prevention of chemotherapy-induced nausea and vomiting in
    patients receiving multiple-day cisplatin chemotherapy for germ cell cancer. Support Care
    Cancer 15:1293–1300
44. Albany C, Brames ML, Fausel C, Johnson CS, Picus J, Einhorn LH (2012) Randomized,
    double-blind, placebo-controlled, phase III crossover study evaluating the oral neurokinin-1
    antagonist aprepitant in combination with a 5-HT3 antagonist plus dexamethasone in patients
    with germ cell tumor receiving 5-day cisplatin combination chemotherapy regimens: a Hoosier
    Oncology Group (HOG) study. J Clin Oncol 30:3998–4003
45. NCCN Clinical Practice Guidelines in Oncology version 1 2015. Antiemesis. National
    Comprehensive Cancer Network (NCCN) [online]. Available from url: http://www.nccn.org/
    professionals/physician_gls/PDF/antiemesis.pdf. Accessed 30 Sept 2015
46. Generic cost of olanzapine. www.goodrx.com. Accessed Oct 2015
47. Editor, Wholesale cost of fosaprepitant (2015) Med Lett 57:60

Chapter 7
Gabapentin for the Prevention of CINV

Thomas J. Guttuso Jr.

Gabapentin is a gamma-aminobutyric acid (GABA) analogue initially approved by the Food and Drug Administration (FDA) in 1993 for the treatment of seizures. Gabapentin was soon found to be highly effective for treating neuropathic pain [1] and then restless legs syndrome [2] and presently is FDA approved for all three indications. Despite its chemical structure, gabapentin has no effect on GABA receptors or GABA breakdown by GABA transaminase but does increase brain GABA synthesis in rats and humans [3, 4]. Gabapentin's mechanism of action for treating neuropathic pain, which is its main clinical use, is dependent upon its binding to the alpha-2/delta subunit of neuronal voltage-gated calcium channels [5] and likely involves the mitigation of neuronal calcium currents [6, 7].

Subsequently, gabapentin was discovered by accident to have two other clinical uses: the treatment of hot flashes and the treatment of chemotherapy-induced nausea and vomiting (CINV).

The discovery of gabapentin for treating hot flashes, also known as vasomotor symptoms (VMS), occurred when a woman who had recently discontinued her hormone replacement therapy (HRT) was placed on gabapentin for migraine prophylaxis and experienced almost complete resolution of her VMS within a few days of initiating gabapentin [8]. This discovery led to several randomized controlled trials (RCTs) that confirmed gabapentin to be an effective VMS therapy [9].

The discovery of gabapentin as a potential, novel anti-nausea and anti-emetic therapy also occurred by accident as an evolution of its use for VMS [10]. A woman with breast cancer was required to discontinue HRT and began experiencing bothersome VMS. She also began four cycles of chemotherapy with doxorubicin 60 mg/m^2 and cyclophosphamide 600 mg/m^2, each round separated by 3 weeks. Ondansetron 10 mg and dexamethasone 10 mg were given before each treatment.

T.J. Guttuso Jr., MD
Department of Neurology, University at Buffalo,
The State University of New York, Buffalo, USA
e-mail: tguttuso@buffalo.edu

© Springer International Publishing Switzerland 2016
R.M. Navari (ed.), *Management of Chemotherapy-Induced Nausea
and Vomiting: New Agents and New Uses of Current Agents*,
DOI 10.1007/978-3-319-27016-6_7

121

The patient reported severe nausea after the first two chemotherapy treatments. Prochlorperazine 10 mg taken 3×/day, as needed, was ineffective. Midway between the second and third chemotherapy treatments, oral gabapentin 300 mg, 3×/day, was started for treatment of the patient's VMS. Within 2 days, all such symptoms had resolved. Unexpectedly, she had no nausea after either the third or the fourth chemotherapy treatments. No other medication changes had been made.

Encouraged by this anecdotal case, we performed an open-label study examining the effects of oral gabapentin 300 mg, 3×/day, on delayed chemotherapy-induced nausea in women with breast cancer who had not previously received chemotherapy [10]. Delayed chemotherapy-induced nausea (days 2–5 after chemotherapy administration) remains a problem for about half of patients receiving moderately emetogenic chemotherapy, despite preventive treatment with a serotonin antagonist and dexamethasone [11]. We screened 21 consecutive patients in a single cancer treatment center and enrolled the first 9 who had experienced at least a moderate degree of delayed chemotherapy-induced nausea after administration of the first of four cycles of adjuvant therapy with doxorubicin 60 mg/m^2 and cyclophosphamide 600 mg/m^2, each cycle separated by 3 weeks. A moderate degree of nausea was defined as a score of 4 or greater on an 8-point nausea scale ("0" being no nausea at all, "1" being mild nausea, and "7" being severe nausea). Subjects recorded a nausea score 4×/day, every 6 h.

For the nine enrolled subjects, gabapentin 300 mg capsules were provided for chemotherapy treatments number 2 and 4 but not for treatments 1 and 3. Gabapentin dosing began 5 days before chemotherapy with one capsule at bedtime for 2 days, then twice daily for 2 days, followed by 3×/day for 6 days, and was discontinued on the sixth day after chemotherapy. All patients received intravenous ondansetron 16–24 mg and intravenous dexamethasone 20 mg with or without intravenous lorazepam 0.5–1.0 mg before all four chemotherapy treatments. Rescue therapy for all treatments consisted of ondansetron 8 mg, 3×/day; prochlorperazine 10 mg, 4×/day; or dexamethasone 20 mg once daily, either alone or in combination and all taken orally, on an as-needed basis. The number of antiemetic pills taken for rescue therapy was also recorded on the nausea diary form for days 1–5 after each chemotherapy treatment. If a patient on gabapentin 300 mg, 3×/day (with no gabapentin-induced side effects) still had nausea after the second chemotherapy treatment, a higher dose of gabapentin, 600 mg, 3×/day, was offered for the fourth chemotherapy treatment. Adverse events were monitored by inquiry during telephone conversations with the patients.

The results showed six of the nine subjects experienced at least a 3-point improvement in peak, delayed nausea on the 8-point scale. Three of these six patients had 6–7 grade, peak delayed nausea during the first cycle of chemotherapy and 0 grade, peak delayed nausea when taking gabapentin for chemotherapy cycles 2 and 4. These improvements were seen despite a median 37 % decrease in the use of prn antiemetics during cycles 2 and 4 when gabapentin was being taken. Two subjects reported mild-moderate drowsiness when taking gabapentin that did not require any dosing adjustments. Figure 7.1 summarizes the median peak nausea data for all nine subjects across the four rounds of chemotherapy.

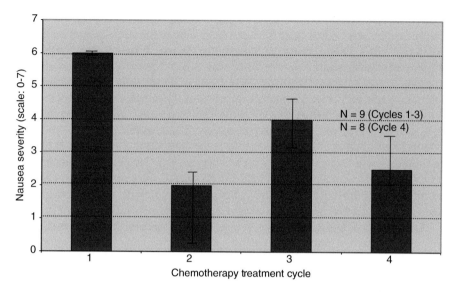

Fig. 7.1 Median peak delayed nausea and interquartile range with gabapentin (cycles 2 and 4) and without gabapentin (cycles 1 and 3)

It is known that patients who experience moderate-severe acute CIN (experienced within the first 24 h after chemotherapy) are not only more likely to experience delayed CIN but are also more resistant to treatments for delayed nausea than are patients with mild acute nausea [12, 13]. In this open-label gabapentin study, eight of the nine subjects experienced moderate-severe acute CIN after their first cycle of chemotherapy when not taking gabapentin. Therefore, 89 % of the subjects enrolled in this study represented those most refractory to conventional antiemetic therapies.

We theorized that gabapentin's mechanism of action in treating chemotherapy-induced delayed nausea might involve decreased tachykinin neurotransmitter activity in relevant brainstem sites such as the area postrema or the nucleus solitarius [10, 14]. It was postulated that this effect may be realized through gabapentin's binding to its principle binding site, the alpha-2/delta subunit of neuronal voltage-gated calcium channels (VGCCs), that had been upregulated on tachykinin neurons in these brainstem sites in response to chemotherapy administration. This upregulation would be expected to markedly increase calcium currents in these neurons [15], which could then increase tachykinin neurotransmitter release and engender clinical nausea and vomiting. There is much evidence that tachykinin activity is involved in the pathogenesis of chemotherapy-induced emesis in ferrets, and a selective tachykinin receptor antagonist improves both acute and delayed nausea and emesis induced by chemotherapy in humans [16].

Such a site-specific upregulation of the alpha-2/delta subunit in response to an environmental stressor has been previously demonstrated in a rat model of neuropathic pain, which is gabapentin's main clinical use. In this neuropathic pain animal model, the environmental stressor was ligation of the sciatic nerve [17]. This study showed a dramatic 17-fold increase in the expression of the alpha-2/delta subunit in the dorsal root ganglia serving the ligated sciatic nerve. It took 7 days for the full 17-fold increase to occur; however, there were two and sevenfold increases already apparent 1 and 2 days after sciatic nerve ligation, respectively. This upregulation and subsequent normalization in the expression of this subunit corresponded to the onset and resolution of behavioral allodynia displayed by the rats, implying that this upregulation is involved in the pathophysiology of neuropathic pain.

It is known that binding of gabapentin to the alpha-2/delta subunit is critical to gabapentin's mechanism of action for treating neuropathic pain. Gabapentin and pregabalin, another high-affinity alpha-2/delta ligand, show no behavioral benefit on allodynia in the mutant, "ducky" strain of mice expressing an altered alpha-2/delta protein for which gabapentin and pregabalin have very little affinity [5].

After publication of the initial report associating gabapentin therapy with reduced delayed CIN, several other groups performed RCTs, examining gabapentin's effects on CINV as well as other clinical conditions associated with nausea and vomiting, primarily postoperative nausea and vomiting (PONV) [18]. In total, there have been nine RCTs (six for PONV, two for CINV, and one for postdural puncture emesis) as well as four case series/reports published to date as full-length manuscripts assessing gabapentin's effects on nausea and vomiting as primary outcome measures (Table 7.1).

As shown in Table 7.1, all six RCTs assessing the effects of a single preoperative gabapentin dose on PONV showed gabapentin to significantly reduce postoperative nausea and 4/6 showed gabapentin to significantly reduce postoperative vomiting. Although PONV is not the topic for this chapter, the design of these trials raises some important points regarding gabapentin dosing that deserve attention.

Administration of an adequate gabapentin dose appears to be critical for its efficacy to be demonstrated across many indications. For example, a daily dose of 300 mg was ineffective for treating hot flashes in postmenopausal women, while 900 mg was effective compared to placebo [30], and 2,400 mg showed efficacy equivalent to high-dose hormone replacement therapy [31], the gold standard therapy for this indication. For the indications of neuropathic pain [32] and restless legs syndrome [2], the gabapentin daily dose demonstrating maximum efficacy is about 1,800–3,600 mg. Such high doses are likely required to achieve maximum clinical efficacy across a population due to the highly variable bioavailability of oral gabapentin, with some subjects absorbing as little as 5 % and some as much as 75 % of a single oral dose [33].

Besides administering an adequate daily dose, the frequency of gabapentin dosing is also important in order to maintain steady serum levels necessary to demonstrate continuous efficacy for long-lasting clinical symptoms. Gabapentin's serum half-life is about 6 h, necessitating 3–4×/day dosing to achieve 24-h symptomatic coverage. These pharmacokinetic features of gabapentin do not appear to have been considered when determining gabapentin dosing for the PONV trials. These trials administered a single 300–600 mg dose 1–2 h before surgery and then assessed N/V for at least the first 24 h after surgery (Table 7.1). In order to achieve symptomatic benefit for 24 h, at least two additional doses of gabapentin would need to have been

Table 7.1 Summary of 13 clinical studies assessing gabapentin's effects on N/V as 1° outcome measures

Study authors	1° outcome measure	Gabapentin dose	Study type	Results
Jahromi et al. (2013) [19]	PONV (facial trauma surgery)	300 mg, 1 h. before IOA	RCT ($n=150$)	Decreased N&V ($p<0.05$)
Misra et al. (2013) [20]	PONV (intracranial surgery)	600 mg, 2 h. before IOA	RCT ($n=73$)	Decreased N ($p=0.02$), not V ($p=0.06$)
Ajori et al. (2012) [21]	PONV (abdominal hysterectomy)	600 mg, 1 h. before IOA	RCT ($n=140$)	Decreased N ($p=0.018$) & V ($p=0.009$)
Khademi et al. (2010) [22]	PONV (open cholecystectomy)	600 mg, 2 h. before IOA	RCT ($n=90$)	Decreased N&V ($p=0.02$)
Mohammadi and Seyedi (2008) [23]	PONV (pelvic lap. surgery)	300 mg, 1 h. before IOA	RCT ($n=70$)	Decreased N ($p=0.022$), not V ($p=0.114$)
Pandey et al. (2006) [24]	PONV (lap. cholecystectomy)	600 mg, 2 h. before IOA	RCT ($n=250$)	Decreased N&V ($p=0.04$)
Guttuso et al. (2005) [25]	PONV (intracranial surgery)	300 mg tid	Case report ($n=1$)	Fully resolved severe emesis and anorexia
Barton et al. (2014) [26]	CINV	300 mg bid	RCT ($n=430$)	Full protection from delayed V and rescue medication use ($p=0.23$)
Cruz et al. (2012) [27]	CINV	300 mg tid	RCT ($n=80$)	Full protection from N&V ($p=0.04$)
Guttuso et al. (2003) [10]	CINV	300 mg tid	Case series ($n=9$)	6/9 of subjects had improved delayed nausea
Guttuso et al. (2010) [14]	HG	1200–3000 mg/day	Case series ($n=7$)	80 % decrease N, 94 % decrease V
Spiegel and Webb (2012) [28]	HG	300 mg tid	Case report ($n=1$)	Decreased PUQE from 15 to 8
Erol (2011) [29]	Postdural puncture headache and emesis	300 mg tid	RCT ($n=42$)	Decreased emesis ($p=0.01$)

PONV postoperative nausea and vomiting, *IOA* induction of anesthesia, *RCT* randomized controlled trial, *N* nausea, *V* vomiting, *lap* laparoscopic, *CINV* chemotherapy-induced nausea and vomiting, *tid* 3×/day, *HG* hyperemesis gravidarum, *PUQE* pregnancy-unique quantification of emesis and nausea

administered based on gabapentin's serum half-life. Despite these oversights, a single preoperative gabapentin dose still provided significant protection from PONV. This is most likely due to the fact that most PONV resolves within 24 h postoperatively.

On the other hand, use of an adequate gabapentin dose administered at least 3×/ day would likely be critical in order to properly assess gabapentin's efficacy in treating delayed CINV since these symptoms persist for about 5 days after chemotherapy administration. In the initial open-label gabapentin pilot study, 7/9 of the subjects experienced adequate subjective benefit from a dose of 300 mg tid while 2/9 of the subjects requested to increase the dose to 600 mg tid for the final round of chemotherapy. This dosing is in concert with what has been effective for other clinical uses of gabapentin, such as VMS, neuropathic pain, and restless legs syndrome [2, 30, 32, 34]. Thus, a minimum dose of 300 mg tid would be recommended for use in CINV trials.

To date, there have been two double-blinded RCTs published as full-length manuscripts assessing gabapentin's effects on CINV. The first by Cruz et al. randomized 80 patients to gabapentin or placebo therapy who were scheduled to receive their first cycle of moderately to highly emetogenic chemotherapy (defined as doses of cisplatin or doxorubicin equal to or greater than 60 and 50 mg/m^2, respectively) [27]. The study capsules were started 5 days prior to chemotherapy administration and slowly titrated to a gabapentin dose of 300 mg tid or matching placebo from the day before to 5 days after chemotherapy. This was the same titration schedule previously used by Guttuso et al. that was shown to be well tolerated [10]. About 91 % of the subjects had breast cancer and received doxorubicin. All subjects also received intravenous ondansetron 8 mg, dexamethasone 10 mg and ranitidine 50 mg before chemotherapy on day 1, and oral dexamethasone 4 mg twice a day on days 2 and 3. Subjects recorded nausea scores and vomiting and retching episodes every day on diary cards as well as the use of rescue antiemetics. The two primary endpoints were complete protection from all nausea and vomiting and no use of rescue medications for days 1–5 and complete protection for days 2–5.

The results showed gabapentin therapy to lead to significantly greater rates of complete protection for days 1–5 ($p = 0.04$) but not for days 2–5 ($p = 0.06$) compared to placebo therapy. Complete protection for days 1–5 occurred in 65 % of subjects taking gabapentin compared to 42.5 % of subjects taking placebo. Adverse events were similar between the groups. The authors noted that the complete protection rates for gabapentin (65 %) compared favorably to the complete protection rates seen in a similarly designed RCT for the neurokinin-1 receptor antagonist aprepitant (51 %) [35], an FDA-approved therapy for prevention of delayed CINV. The gabapentin and aprepitant trials had nearly identical placebo arm complete response rates for days 1–5 (42.5 % and 42 %, respectively). The authors suggested that a single trial comparing gabapentin with aprepitant was merited based on their study results and the significant savings that could be achieved by using a generic medication like gabapentin versus aprepitant. This savings has been estimated to be $315–$484/cycle of chemotherapy [18, 27].

A small, open-label, randomized trial directly comparing aprepitant and gabapentin for refractory CINV has been performed but has only been published as an abstract [36]. In this trial, 13 of 77 subjects (17 %) receiving their first cycle of "level 3, 4, or 5" emetogenic-potential chemotherapy required rescue antiemetic therapy despite receiving "standard dexamethasone and ondansetron." These 13 subjects were then randomized to receive either open-label aprepitant (6) or open-label gabapentin (7) during their second cycle of chemotherapy. The aprepitant group received 125 mg on day 1 and 80 mg on days 2 and 3 and the gabapentin group received 300 mg tid for days −2 to 5, with day 1 being the day of chemotherapy administration. Subjects recorded their nausea and vomiting on a "validated" scoring system with 0 being no N/V and 15 being the worst N/V.

The results of this small trial showed mean N/V scores to improve from the first (control) to the second (treatment) chemotherapy cycles from 7.0 to 2.66 for the aprepitant group and from 7.43 to 1.0 for the gabapentin group. There were no differences in toxicity profile and subject-reported satisfaction levels between the two groups. No statistical analyses were reported.

The second CINV trial, by Barton et al., represents the largest RCT performed to date evaluating gabapentin's anti-nausea and antiemetic actions. This study randomized 430 subjects scheduled to receive their first cycle of highly emetogenic chemotherapy to either gabapentin or matching placebo for days 1–5. All subjects also received a serotonin antagonist, like ondansetron, and dexamethasone 20 mg before chemotherapy on day 1 and decreasing doses of oral dexamethasone from days 2–4 (starting at 16 mg a day on day 2). In addition, subjects could also receive a serotonin antagonist on days 2–5 based on the treating physicians' preferences. For this study, in contrast to the three gabapentin CINV trials outlined above, gabapentin/placebo was not started before day 1 but was started on day 1 (after chemotherapy administration) with a single 300 mg bedtime dose and then increased to 300 mg bid for days 2–5. The dose could be increased to tid for days 4–5 if subjects desired based on their symptoms. Subjects recorded nausea scores and vomiting and retching episodes every day on diary cards as well as the use of rescue antiemetics. The Functional Living Index-Emesis (FLIE) [37] and subject satisfaction were also assessed. The primary endpoint was complete protection from all vomiting and use of rescue medications for days 2–6.

The results showed 47 % of subjects in the gabapentin arm and 41 % in the placebo arm had a complete response ($p=0.23$) over days 2–6. Subgroup analyses for each day showed significantly higher rates of complete response for the gabapentin arm on days 2–4 but not for days 5–6. There were no significant intergroup differences on mean number of vomiting episodes, mean nausea scores, mean number of rescue antiemetics, FLIE scores, or subject satisfaction. Thirty percent of subjects in each group experienced vomiting, and 45 % and 53 % of subjects in the gabapentin and placebo arms, respectively, took any rescue antiemetics ($p=0.12$). The percent of subjects choosing to increase their study medication from bid to tid on days 4 or 5 was not significantly different between groups (≤9 % of subjects on day 4 and ≤6 % on day 5). The only side effects that significantly differed between the groups were negative mood swings and appetite loss, both favoring the placebo arm; however, the magnitude of these differences was not felt to be clinically meaningful.

This study also reported subjects' nausea and vomiting data for each day from days 2–6. Mean nausea scores for each group on a scale from 0 to 10 were ≤1.5 for each day and mean number of vomiting episodes were ≤0.3 for each day. Such low levels of nausea and vomiting suggest that these subjects did not experience clinically meaningful symptoms despite receiving highly emetogenic chemotherapy. This observation was further supported by the high levels of health-related quality of life on the FLIE and high satisfaction reported by subjects in both groups. The mean FLIE scores for both groups were >108 (maximum possible score = 126) and mean satisfaction scores were >8.0 (maximum possible score = 10). It is known that a FLIE score of ≥108 indicates no negative impact on daily functioning [38, 39].

There are several methodological features of this study that may have contributed to its negative results; however, the most salient is that the target population, patients with clinically meaningful delayed CINV, was not assessed. It is not clear why this occurred as a previous study showed much lower FLIE scores (mean of 95.5), indicating a meaningful negative impact on daily functioning, for patients receiving highly emetogenic chemotherapy [39]. It is unfortunate that such a large study failed to capture this target population. As a result, no reliable conclusions can be made on gabapentin's effectiveness for preventing CINV based on this study's results. The authors noted this fact and recommended that future trials should not include "all comers" but should focus on the roughly 25 % of patients who experience moderate to severe nausea and emesis that affect their functioning despite receiving evidence-based prophylactic treatment. This recommendation is very appropriate regarding the clinical generalizability of such trials since, in the real-world clinic, most patients would not be offered extra therapy for delayed CINV unless they were felt to need it based on their symptoms from a previous cycle of chemotherapy.

Another methodological feature of this study that may have contributed to the negative results may have been the use of an inadequate dose of gabapentin. Previous trials that had shown more promising results used at least 900 mg/day of gabapentin that was started before day 1 of chemotherapy. In this study, gabapentin was not started until after chemotherapy was administered and 88 % of subjects in the gabapentin arm received a maximum gabapentin dose of only 600 mg/day for days 2–5.

The potential impact of gabapentin dosing on CINV can be seen by comparing the complete responder rates between the Cruz et al. and the Barton et al. trials. In the Cruz et al. trial, gabapentin was initiated on day −5 and slowly titrated up to 900 mg/day by day −1 and continued at that dose through day 5; this trial showed mean complete responder rates of 72.5 % and 52.5 % for the gabapentin and placebo groups, respectively, for days 2–5. In the Barton et al. trial, gabapentin was initiated on day 1 and continued at a dose of 600 mg/day in 88 % of these subjects for days 2–6; this trial showed mean complete responder rates of 47 % and 41 % for the gabapentin and placebo groups, respectively, for days 2–6. Thus, the extra 300 mg/day of gabapentin used in the Cruz et al. trial compared to the Barton et al. trial was associated with a 14 % larger treatment effect size (difference between the gabapentin and placebo arm complete responder rates). Although comparing results between separate trials can lead to flawed conclusions, these results suggest that a minimum gabapentin dose of 900 mg/day should be used in future CINV trials. This dose is also consistent with what has been shown to be the minimum effective gabapentin dose for treating VMS [30]. Furthermore, it is quite possible that gabapentin doses even higher than 900 mg/day would be more effective for CINV based on the doses that have been shown to be most effective for VMS, neuropathic pain, and restless legs syndrome [2, 31, 32].

Upon reviewing the designs and results of the above 4 clinical trials evaluating the effectiveness of gabapentin for preventing delayed CINV, a few recommendations can be made for the design of future trials. First, subjects receiving their first cycle of moderately or highly emetogenic chemotherapy should be screened, and only those with at least a moderate degree of nausea or any vomiting should be randomized to a treatment arm for their second cycle. This will assure that the target population of patients with refractory nausea and vomiting would be studied. Also, requiring the nausea and vomiting symptoms to result in a minimum level of functional impact, such as having a FLIE score of <108, would also be recommended as an inclusion criteria to confirm that the studied population would have clinically meaningful symptoms. Barton et al. estimated that about 25 % of patients screened during their first cycle would satisfy such eligibility criteria [26]. In the pilot study by Guttuso et al. 9 out of 21 consecutive patients (43 %) screened during their first cycle of moderately emetogenic chemotherapy experienced at least a moderate level of delayed CIN [10]. On the other hand, Pacheco et al. found only 17 % of patients required rescue antiemetic therapy after their first cycle of moderately to highly emetogenic chemotherapy.

Another methodological issue that deserves attention is the choice of primary endpoint. By convention, most CINV clinical trials have used complete responder rate as the primary endpoint. A complete response is typically defined as not experiencing any vomiting or use of rescue antiemetics. Such a focus on vomiting may not be an appropriate primary endpoint when considering the chemotherapy-associated symptoms most meaningful to patients.

A study performed in 1993 among 155 cancer patients who had received chemotherapy within the previous 4 weeks showed that subjects reported nausea as the most severe and troublesome symptom experienced from chemotherapy followed by tiredness and hair loss [40]. This research team had performed this same study in 1983. The most marked change from 1983 to 1993 was subjects' rating of vomiting severity, which was rated as the most severe symptom in 1983 but dropped to the fifth most severe symptom in 1993. In the subgroup of patients >60 years old, vomiting was rated as the 15th most severe symptom in 1993. The researches attributed this drop in vomiting severity to the standard use in 1993 of serotonin antagonists, high-dose metoclopramide, and steroids that were not widely used in 1983. A more recent study among 298 cancer patients receiving moderately or highly emetogenic chemotherapy confirmed that nausea contributed more to reduced quality of life than did vomiting as measured by the FLIE [39].

Furthermore, the Barton et al. study showed that subjects randomized to placebo therapy were not negatively impacted by their chemotherapy based on this group's mean FLIE score of 108.5. Nevertheless, this group had a complete response rate of only 41 % for days 2–6 [26]. Thus, almost 60 % of subjects were "treatment failures," based on the primary endpoint definition; however, this treatment failure status was not at all reflected in the mean FLIE scores. One explanation for this disparity may be due to the failure of the primary end point to reflect the most severe and meaningful symptom for chemotherapy patients, nausea, while the FLIE reflected the functional impact of both nausea and vomiting symptoms.

Thus, a more appropriate primary assessment of a meaningful CINV therapy in modern times would need to include a nausea assessment. Since CIN is much less likely to fully resolve than CIV, it would be logical to include two co-primary end points for future CINV trials: (1) complete response rates and (2) hours/day of nausea. In another patient population, the number of hours of nausea/day has been found to be a more accurate indicator of nausea impact than nausea severity assessments [41]. A therapy would need to show significant benefits for both endpoints against a comparison arm in order to be considered more effective.

In terms of secondary endpoints, in addition to a functional outcome, such as the FLIE, another very useful secondary endpoint would be to assess subjects' global satisfaction of treatment on a 7-point Likert scale and compare "global satisfaction responder rates," defined as the % of subjects recording a 6 or 7, between the groups. One of the main benefits of assessing global satisfaction is that it is a comprehensive assessment that encompasses both a treatment's benefits and side effects and their magnitude of subjective impact all in a single assessment. The global satisfaction responder rates may also better reflect a therapy's utility in the real-world clinic compared to a narrow focus on a therapy's benefit for only one symptom [42]. In addition to the FLIE and global satisfaction assessments, an assessment of fatigue, such as the fatigue severity scale [43], would be indicated considering that cancer patients report fatigue as the second most severe symptom associated with chemotherapy [40].

7.1 Conclusion

The evidence to date supports gabapentin to potentially be an effective therapy for delayed CINV, but further well-designed RCTs are clearly needed. The two gabapentin trials that utilized the important methodology of screening patients and only enrolling those with refractory delayed CINV unfortunately were both unblinded, open-label trials [10, 36]. Nevertheless, both of these small trials showed very promising results, especially the Pacheco et al. trial that showed subjects randomized to gabapentin to have an absolute 25 % greater reduction in mean N/V scores from baseline as subjects randomized to aprepitant. One of the two double-blinded, RCTs showed gabapentin to be more effective than placebo [27]; however, the other did not [26]. Unfortunately, both of these trials failed to screen patients for refractory delayed CINV, which resulted in subjects having fairly minor N/V symptoms in both study arms, especially for the Barton et al. trial. Thus, the question of whether gabapentin is effective for delayed CINV in patients refractory to serotonin antagonists and steroids remains unanswered.

The NK-1 antagonist aprepitant is currently FDA approved for delayed CINV; however, its use may be limited mostly due to its high cost but also due to its potential for drug-drug interactions from its metabolism by the P450 enzyme system, specifically CYP3A4 [26]. Nevertheless, as aprepitant is FDA approved and widely available, it would be unethical to design a placebo-controlled trial among patients with refractory delayed CINV, which would deny 50 % of the subjects from receiving a standard of care therapy. Barton et al. noted this ethical issue as a primary reason for their trial design to include "all comers."

Now, with data from four gabapentin CINV trials providing a signal that gabapentin may be as effective and possibly even more effective than aprepitant for delayed CINV, a comparative trial directly comparing the two compounds is merited [27, 35, 36]. Such a trial is further justified due to the potential for significant cost savings and the absence of significant drug-drug interactions [44] with gabapentin compared to aprepitant.

The ideal trial design would be a double-blind, randomized trial among subjects experiencing at least moderate delayed nausea and some vomiting despite receiving a serotonin antagonist and steroids with their first cycle of moderately to highly emetogenic chemotherapy. These subjects with refractory delayed CINV would then be randomized to gabapentin or aprepitant treatment for their second cycle of chemotherapy in addition to the same standard antiemetic therapy they received with their first chemotherapy cycle. There would be two co-primary endpoints of (1) rates of complete response and (2) hours/day of any nausea. Secondary endpoints would include FLIE scores, fatigue severity scores, and global satisfaction scores. The study capsules would be started 5 days before chemotherapy and slowly titrated up to 1 capsule qid for days 1–5, which would be a gabapentin dose of 300 mg qid for days 1–5 or an aprepitant dose of 125 mg on day 1 and 80 mg qAM on days 2–3. The slightly higher dose of gabapentin compared to those used in previous CINV trials would be warranted to better assure maximum efficacy based on the gabapentin doses shown to have maximum efficacy for other indications [2, 31, 32, 34].

References

1. Backonja M, Beydoun A, Edwards KR et al (1998) Gabapentin for the symptomatic treatment of painful neuropathy in patients with diabetes mellitus: a randomized controlled trial. JAMA 280:1831–1836
2. Garcia-Borreguero D, Larrosa O, de la Llave Y, Verger K, Masramon X, Hernandez G (2002) Treatment of restless legs syndrome with gabapentin: a double-blind, cross-over study. Neurology 59:1573–1579
3. Chadwick D (1992) Gabapentin. In: Pedley TA, Meldrum BS (eds) Recent advances in epilepsy. Churchill-Livingstone, Edinburgh, pp 211–221
4. Taylor CP (1997) Mechanisms of action of gabapentin. Rev Neurol (Paris) 153(Suppl 1):S39–S45
5. Taylor CP (2004) The biology and pharmacology of calcium channel (alpha)2(delta) proteins. Pfizer satellite symposium to the 2003 Society for Neuroscience Meeting. Sheraton New Orleans Hotel, New Orleans, LA November 10, 2003. CNS Drug Rev 10:183–188
6. Fink K, Dooley DJ, Meder WP et al (2002) Inhibition of neuronal Ca(2+) influx by gabapentin and pregabalin in the human neocortex. Neuropharmacology 42:229–236
7. Sutton KG, Martin DJ, Pinnock RD, Lee K, Scott RH (2002) Gabapentin inhibits high-threshold calcium channel currents in cultured rat dorsal root ganglion neurones. Br J Pharmacol 135:257–265

8. Guttuso TJ Jr (2000) Gabapentin's effects on hot flashes and hypothermia. Neurology 54:2161–2163
9. Guttuso T Jr (2012) Effective and clinically meaningful non-hormonal hot flash therapies. Maturitas 72:6–12
10. Guttuso T Jr, Roscoe J, Griggs J (2003) Effect of gabapentin on nausea induced by chemotherapy in patients with breast cancer. Lancet 361:1703–1705
11. Pater JL, Lofters WS, Zee B et al (1997) The role of the 5-HT3 antagonists ondansetron and dolasetron in the control of delayed onset nausea and vomiting in patients receiving moderately emetogenic chemotherapy. Ann Oncol 8:181–185
12. Dexamethasone alone or in combination with ondansetron for the prevention of delayed nausea and vomiting induced by chemotherapy. The Italian Group for Antiemetic Research (2000) N Engl J Med 342:1554–1559
13. Kris MG, Gralla RJ, Clark RA et al (1985) Incidence, course, and severity of delayed nausea and vomiting following the administration of high-dose cisplatin. J Clin Oncol 3:1379–1384
14. Guttuso T Jr, Robinson LK, Amankwah KS (2010) Gabapentin use in hyperemesis gravidarum: a pilot study. Early Hum Dev 86:65–66
15. Shistik E, Ivanina T, Puri T, Hosey M, Dascal N (1995) Ca2+ current enhancement by alpha 2/delta and beta subunits in Xenopus oocytes: contribution of changes in channel gating and alpha 1 protein level. J Physiol 489:55–62
16. Navari RM, Reinhardt RR, Gralla RJ et al (1999) Reduction of cisplatin-induced emesis by a selective neurokinin-1-receptor antagonist. L-754,030 Antiemetic Trials Group. N Engl J Med 340:190–195
17. Luo ZD, Chaplan SR, Higuera ES et al (2001) Upregulation of dorsal root ganglion (alpha)2(delta) calcium channel subunit and its correlation with allodynia in spinal nerve-injured rats. J Neurosci 21:1868–1875
18. Guttuso T Jr (2014) Gabapentin's anti-nausea and anti-emetic effects: a review. Exp Brain Res 232:2535–2539
19. Jahromi HE, Gholami M, Rezaei F (2013) A randomized double-blinded placebo controlled study of four interventions for the prevention of postoperative nausea and vomiting in maxillofacial trauma surgery. J Craniofac Surg 24:e623–e627
20. Misra S, Parthasarathi G, Vilanilam GC (2013) The effect of gabapentin premedication on postoperative nausea, vomiting, and pain in patients on preoperative dexamethasone undergoing craniotomy for intracranial tumors. J Neurosurg Anesthesiol 25:386–391
21. Ajori L, Nazari L, Mazloomfard MM, Amiri Z (2012) Effects of gabapentin on postoperative pain, nausea and vomiting after abdominal hysterectomy: a double blind randomized clinical trial. Arch Gynecol Obstet 285:677–682
22. Khademi S, Ghaffarpasand F, Heiran HR, Asefi A (2010) Effects of preoperative gabapentin on postoperative nausea and vomiting after open cholecystectomy: a prospective randomized double-blind placebo-controlled study. Med Princ Pract 19:57–60
23. Mohammadi SS, Seyedi M (2008) Effects of gabapentin on early postoperative pain, nausea and vomiting in laparoscopic surgery for assisted reproductive technologies. Pak J Biol Sci: PJBS 11:1878–1880
24. Pandey CK, Priye S, Ambesh SP, Singh S, Singh U, Singh PK (2006) Prophylactic gabapentin for prevention of postoperative nausea and vomiting in patients undergoing laparoscopic cholecystectomy: a randomized, double-blind, placebo-controlled study. J Postgrad Med 52:97–100
25. Guttuso T Jr, Vitticore P, Holloway RG (2005) Responsiveness of life-threatening refractory emesis to gabapentin-scopolamine therapy following posterior fossa surgery. Case Rep J Neurosurg 102:547–549
26. Barton DL, Thanarajasingam G, Sloan JA et al (2014) Phase III double-blind, placebo-controlled study of gabapentin for the prevention of delayed chemotherapy-induced nausea and vomiting in patients receiving highly emetogenic chemotherapy. NCCTG N08C3 (Alliance). Cancer

27. Cruz FM, de Iracema Gomes Cubero D, Taranto P et al (2012) Gabapentin for the prevention of chemotherapy- induced nausea and vomiting: a pilot study. Support Care Cancer 20:601–606

28. Spiegel DR, Webb K (2012) A case of treatment refractory hyperemesis gravidarum in a patient with comorbid anxiety, treated successfully with adjunctive gabapentin: a review and the potential role of neurogastroentereology in understanding its pathogenesis and treatment. Innov Clin Neurosci 9:31–38

29. Erol DD (2011) The analgesic and antiemetic efficacy of gabapentin or ergotamine/caffeine for the treatment of postdural puncture headache. Adv Med Sci 56:25–29

30. Pandya KJ, Morrow GR, Roscoe JA et al (2005) Gabapentin for hot flashes in 420 women with breast cancer: a randomised double-blind placebo-controlled trial. Lancet 366:818–824

31. Reddy SY, Warner H, Guttuso T Jr et al (2006) Gabapentin, estrogen, and placebo for treating hot flushes: a randomized controlled trial. Obstet Gynecol 108:41–48

32. Backonja M, Glanzman RL (2003) Gabapentin dosing for neuropathic pain: evidence from randomized, placebo-controlled clinical trials. Clin Ther 25:81–104

33. AGidal BE, Radulovic LL, Kruger S, Rutecki P, Pitterle M, Bockbrader HN (2000) Inter- and intra-subject variability in gabapentin absorption and absolute bioavailability. Epilepsy Res 40:123–127

34. Guttuso T Jr, Kurlan R, McDermott MP, Kieburtz K (2003) Gabapentin's effects on hot flashes in postmenopausal women: a randomized controlled trial. Obstet Gynecol 101:337–345

35. Warr DG, Hesketh PJ, Gralla RJ et al (2005) Efficacy and tolerability of aprepitant for the prevention of chemotherapy-induced nausea and vomiting in patients with breast cancer after moderately emetogenic chemotherapy. J Clin Oncol 23:2822–2830

36. Pacheco A, Verschraegen CF, Mangalik A, Cheshire S, Royce ME (2008) A randomized open-label comparison of aprepitant (A) versus gabapentin (G) in the prevention of the refractory nausea and vomiting associated with moderately and severely emetogenic chemotherapy. J Clin Oncol 26(Suppl):20509

37. Martin AR, Pearson JD, Cai B, Elmer M, Horgan K, Lindley C (2003) Assessing the impact of chemotherapy-induced nausea and vomiting on patients' daily lives: a modified version of the Functional Living Index-Emesis (FLIE) with 5-day recall. Support Care Cancer 11:522–527

38. Haiderali A, Menditto L, Good M, Teitelbaum A, Wegner J (2011) Impact on daily functioning and indirect/direct costs associated with chemotherapy-induced nausea and vomiting (CINV) in a U.S. population. Support Care Cancer 19:843–851

39. Bloechl-Daum B, Deuson RR, Mavros P, Hansen M, Herrstedt J (2006) Delayed nausea and vomiting continue to reduce patients' quality of life after highly and moderately emetogenic chemotherapy despite antiemetic treatment. J Clin Oncol 24:4472–4478

40. Griffin AM, Butow PN, Coates AS et al (1996) On the receiving end. V: patient perceptions of the side effects of cancer chemotherapy in 1993. Ann Oncol 7:189–195

41. Koren G, Boskovic R, Hard M, Maltepe C, Navioz Y, Einarson A (2002) Motherisk-PUQE (pregnancy-unique quantification of emesis and nausea) scoring system for nausea and vomiting of pregnancy. Am J Obstet Gynecol 186:S228–S231

42. Pleil AM, Coyne KS, Reese PR, Jumadilova Z, Rovner ES, Kelleher CJ (2005) The validation of patient-rated global assessments of treatment benefit, satisfaction, and willingness to continue – the BSW. Value Health: J Int Soc Pharmacoeconomics Outcome Res 8(Suppl 1):S25–S34

43. Krupp LB, LaRocca NG, Muir-Nash J, Steinberg AD (1989) The fatigue severity scale. Application to patients with multiple sclerosis and systemic lupus erythematosus. Arch Neurol 46:1121–1123

44. Radulovic LL, Turck D, von Hodenberg A et al (1995) Disposition of gabapentin (neurontin) in mice, rats, dogs, and monkeys. Drug Metab Dispos 23:441–448

Chapter 8
Prevention of CINV in Patients Receiving High-Dose Multiple-Day Chemotherapy

Luigi Celio

8.1 Introduction

High-dose chemotherapy involves the administration of extremely high, potentially toxic, doses of chemotherapeutic agents in an effort to eradicate cancer cells. A wide range of high-dose regimens has been developed, and they typically consist of several agents given at high doses over 2–7 days [1–3]. Myeloablative chemotherapy is usually followed by a bone marrow or peripheral blood stem-cell transplantation to rebuild the bone marrow. Allogeneic hematopoietic stem-cell transplantation (allo-HSCT) is a potentially curative treatment modality for many hematological malignancies [4]. Following a preparative regimen (i.e., the conditioning), the patient receives stem cells from an unrelated or related donor to replace their own hematopoietic system [5]. In allo-HSCT, classic myeloablative conditioning consists of high-dose chemotherapy with or without total body irradiation (TBI). In the past two decades, peripheral blood stem cells replaced bone marrow as stem-cell source due to faster engraftment and practicability [5]. The use of peripheral blood as a source of stem cells for autologous HSCT (auto-HSCT) greatly contributed to the application of high-dose chemotherapy in the treatment of both hematological and solid malignancies [3, 6, 7]. In auto-HSCT, patients receive their own stem cells, and this has the advantage of lower risk of infection, since the recovery of immune function is rapid.

All high-dose chemotherapy regimens are associated with significant acute and late toxicities. Severe neutropenia, thrombocytopenia, and anemia are the main causes of acute hematological toxicity which leads to the necessity of transfusion

L. Celio, MD
Department of Medical Oncology 1, Fondazione IRCCS Istituto Nazionale Tumori,
Via G. Venezian 1, Milan 20133, Italy
e-mail: luigi.celio@istitutotumori.mi.it

© Springer International Publishing Switzerland 2016
R.M. Navari (ed.), *Management of Chemotherapy-Induced Nausea and Vomiting: New Agents and New Uses of Current Agents*,
DOI 10.1007/978-3-319-27016-6_8

support and an increased risk of febrile neutropenia and sepsis [8]. Acute non-hematological toxicities include nausea, vomiting, diarrhea, fatigue, and mucositis.

During the past two decades, major advances have been made in the control of chemotherapy-induced nausea and vomiting (CINV) caused by conventional-dose chemotherapy [9]. The improvements have been achieved through well-designed and adequately powered controlled trials that established the value of modern anti-emetics such as 5-hydroxytryptamine type-3 (5-HT$_3$) receptor antagonists and neu-rokinin-1 (NK-1) receptor antagonists in the prevention of acute- and delayed-onset CINV. Unfortunately, there has been only limited progress in the prevention of CINV caused by high-dose chemotherapy. In this chapter, I provide an overview of CINV in patients undergoing high-dose chemotherapy regimens, with a focus on challenges and unmet needs in this special population. I also provide an overview of the results with modern antiemetics in this setting. Finally, current treatment guide-lines are also discussed along with suggestions for future investigations.

8.2   CINV in Patients Undergoing High-Dose Chemotherapy

In the setting of high-dose chemotherapy with HSCT, nausea and vomiting are almost universal and can have profound clinical and psychological implications for the patient [10]. Although some patient-related characteristics are well-known risk factors for CINV, the intrinsic emetogenicity of a given chemotherapeutic agent as well as its potential to induce acute or delayed emesis should serve as the main fac-tors in guiding preventive strategies for CINV [9]. In addition, chemotherapeutic agents such as cyclophosphamide, carboplatin, cytarabine, and melphalan may be of moderate emetogenic risk when used at conventional doses, but they are highly emetogenic when employed in doses well above the ones conventionally given [9, 11, 12]. Owing to the higher doses of chemotherapy given in preparation for HSCT and to the combinations of agents administered, conditioning regimens have the potential to cause more nausea and vomiting, especially with regard to delayed symptoms, than commonly used high-dose cisplatin. In the HSCT setting, nausea and vomiting may occur during administration of anticancer agents, and delayed symptoms may also occur for days or weeks during the recovery period from sys-temic chemotherapy [10, 13]. In addition, TBI used in many conditioning regimens is associated with a number of acute side effects that include nausea and vomiting, compounding the side effects of high-dose chemotherapy [14]. In spite of the widely held assumption that cancer patients undergoing high-dose chemotherapy experi-ence nausea and vomiting that are more severe than those with conventional-dose chemotherapy, there are few published data concerning both the natural history of emesis in this special population and the severity of delayed symptoms [10, 15].

A multicenter, prospective, observational study evaluated the incidence and sever-ity of CINV in 100 consecutive transplantation recipients [16]. Twenty-six patients were conditioned with a regimen containing TBI and 74 patients without TBI. The most common chemotherapy regimen was busulfan/cyclophosphamide (Bu/CY) used in 29 % of the patients, followed by BCNU/etoposide/ara-C/melphalan (BEAM) in 26 % of the patients. Forty-four patients received an allo-HSCT and 56 patients received an auto-HSCT. While all patients received at least a 5-HT$_3$ receptor antagonist and dopamine antagonists, corticosteroids were not used. In this study, complete response (CR; defined as no vomiting and no rescue antiemetics) occurred only in few patients (19 %) during the 5-day study period after the start of conditioning regimen. In addition, CINV had a deleterious effect on patient's quality of life as assessed through a validated functional living Index-Emesis (FLIE) questionnaire.

A retrospective review evaluated antiemetic outcome in 176 patients admitted to the adult Bone Marrow Unit at Memorial Sloan-Kettering Cancer Center [17]. All patients received a conditioning regimen for which the mean duration was 5 days (range, 1–9 days). Antiemetic prophylaxis consisted of a 5-HT$_3$ receptor antagonist, but dexamethasone was occasionally used when there was no other contraindication to its use with some conditioning regimens. The study showed that auto-HSCT is associated with less nausea and vomiting (51 % and 18 %, respectively) than allo-HSCT (78 % and 39 %, respectively). Patients receiving irradiation had a higher incidence of nausea and vomiting (81 % and 33 %, respectively) compared with those receiving chemotherapy-only conditioning regimens (51 % and 20 %, respectively). Among all disease groups, leukemia patients had the highest incidence of nausea (85 %) and vomiting (45 %).

The above findings support the conclusion that high-dose chemotherapy with HSCT provides a unique challenge to achieving good antiemetic control. In addition to the administration of chemotherapeutic agents at higher doses, a number of potential factors may contribute to an increased incidence and severity of CINV in this setting such as consecutive-day administration, prior treatment with chemotherapy, inclusion of radiation therapy (especially TBI) which increases emetogenic risk, and associated other medical conditions or medications that may cause emesis [2, 13]. Since high-dose chemotherapy is typically administered in a multiple daily-dose schedule, a major problem is the complexity of the emetic stimulus in these patients. The pathophysiology of nausea and vomiting when emetogenic chemotherapy is given over more than 1 day is complicated by the fact that patients can suffer from both acute and delayed nausea and vomiting, and delayed symptoms can continue in the days after chemotherapy completion [18]. Accordingly, nausea and vomiting caused by high-dose chemotherapy worsen progressively with the prolongation of treatment. It also must be pointed out that patients undergoing HSCT have often been heavily pretreated with chemotherapy and, therefore, have varied history of acute and delayed symptoms, anticipatory CINV, and use of different antiemetic regimens [2, 13]. In the posttransplantation period, the risk of delayed nausea and vomiting is also influenced by multiple confounding variables, including damage to the gastrointestinal mucosa, delayed effects of radiation, concomitant administration of intensive prophylaxis or treatment with emetogenic intravenous antimicrobials and antifungals, and use of narcotic analgesics to manage mucositis, profound neutropenia, and immunosuppressive agents [14]. High-dose chemotherapy alone or in combination with TBI prior to HSCT causes significant and prolonged (from days to weeks) disruption of gastrointestinal lining, a late event that may result in continual source of both serotonin and substance P (SP) release [2]. Serotonin that mainly stimulates the 5-HT$_3$ receptors on the vagal afferent fibers located in the gastrointestinal tract and SP, the endogenous ligand acting preferentially on NK-1 receptors located in the brain, may serve as a constant stimulus to nausea and vomiting. It also should be noted that the cryopreservative dimethyl sulfoxide in which stem cells have been suspended is itself emetogenic when reinfused [19]. Therefore, it may be a very hard task to evaluate the efficacy of antiemetic strategies during the posttransplantation period due to so many confounding factors. In order to circumvent these pitfalls, it has been suggested that the design of an ideal study assessing antiemetic outcome during high-dose chemotherapy with HSCT should include only patients undergoing the same preparative regimen and the same type of transplantation [13]. The trial should not include patients with a history of anticipatory CINV and also control for the use of extra steroids beyond those that may be included in the antiemetic regimens employed. The trial should also consider the effects of other medications on the rising incidence of nausea and vomiting that may be observed on the day of the transplantation and the following days.

8.3   First-Generation 5-HT$_3$ Receptor Antagonists for High-Dose Chemotherapy

One of the most significant advances in the management of acute CINV has been the introduction of selective 5-HT$_3$ receptor antagonists, namely, ondansetron, granisetron, dolasetron, and tropisetron [9]. Outside of the HSCT setting, randomized trials have demonstrated the therapeutic equivalence of the first-generation antagonists, a finding supported by a number of meta-analyses [20, 21]. While in patients undergoing high-dose chemotherapy with HSCT, the majority of reports have been published as single-arm trials to assess antiemetic outcome of a 5-HT$_3$ receptor antagonist alone or combined with dexamethasone; limited data from studies directly comparing these agents are available [15].

A single-center, small-size study compared the efficacy of three 5-HT$_3$ receptor antagonists during the conditioning for auto-HSCT [22]. Forty-five patients suffering from malignant lymphoma who were scheduled to receive BEAM chemotherapy as conditioning prior to HSCT were randomized to receive one of three antiemetic agents: granisetron 3 mg intravenously once a day, tropisetron 5 mg intravenously once a day, or ondansetron 8 mg intravenously twice daily on each day of the conditioning. Antiemetic control failure was defined as nausea lasting ≥ 4 h and/or ≥ 3 episodes of vomiting on each single day of the study period. The three 5-HT$_3$ receptor antagonists sufficiently controlled nausea and vomiting in 67–87 % of the patients during the 6-day chemotherapy period. In the overall study period (10 days), both granisetron and tropisetron proved to be more effective in the posttransplantation period, when emetogenic factors other than chemotherapy alone may affect the control of emesis.

A double-blind, phase III study evaluated the efficacy of two orally administered 5-HT$_3$ receptor antagonists versus ondansetron intravenously for the prevention of CINV caused by high-dose chemotherapy or chemoradiotherapy prior to auto-HSCT [23]. A total of 102 patients were randomized to receive either oral ondansetron 8 mg three times a day, oral granisetron 1 mg twice daily, or ondansetron 32 mg intravenously once a day on each day of various conditioning regimens plus one additional day. All patients also received dexamethasone 10 mg intravenously once a day while receiving a 5-HT$_3$ receptor antagonist. The most common chemotherapy regimen was cyclophosphamide/thiotepa/carboplatin in 33 % of the patients, followed by etoposide/cyclophosphamide with TBI in 26 % of the patients. There were no statistically significant differences in the rates of overall CR (defined as none-to-mild nausea and no rescue antiemetics) among the three antiemetic regimens (48 % vs. 47 % vs. 49 %, respectively, for oral ondansetron, oral granisetron, and bolus ondansetron).

A prospective, randomized study compared the efficacy of granisetron and dexamethasone to that of granisetron alone for the prevention of CINV in patients receiving high-dose chemotherapy with or without TBI prior to HSCT [24]. Patients were randomized to receive granisetron 40 µg/kg intravenously twice daily with or without 4 mg dexamethasone just before each dose of chemotherapeutic agent or TBI or 12 h after the first dose if TBI or a drug was given once a day. Fifty patients were evaluable for the analysis. During the first 24 h of conditioning, 92 % of the patients in the granisetron-plus-dexamethasone arm achieved complete control (CC) of emesis (defined as no emetic episodes over the course of a day), compared with 72 % in the granisetron-alone arm. For patients receiving TBI on the first day of conditioning, CC of emesis was achieved in all patients in the granisetron-plus-dexamethasone arm compared with 63 % in the granisetron-alone arm. The same degree of emetic control was maintained throughout the conditioning period in 39 % of the patients in the two-drug combination arm and 30 % of the patients who received granisetron alone. These findings suggested that granisetron in combination with dexamethasone is superior to granisetron alone for the prevention of emesis resulting from the conditioning.

In a double-blind, randomized trial, the comparative efficacy of ondansetron and granisetron was evaluated during conditioning prior to HSCT [25]. Patients were randomized to receive either ondansetron 0.15 mg/kg intravenously three times a day or granisetron 10 µg/kg intravenously once a day. Additionally, all patients received scheduled dexamethasone and lorazepam. Antiemetic prophylaxis was continued until 24 h after chemotherapy completion. In this study, there were patients with a variety of different malignancies who received a variety of conditioning regimens. Among the 110 randomized patients, 96 were evaluable for efficacy within 1 week of study initiation. On day 1, CR (defined as no emetic episodes, and none-to-mild nausea) occurred in 83–90 % of the patients in the two treatment arms, but daily control of emesis decreased, with loss of efficacy for both agents by day 6 after the start of conditioning therapy. On day 6, only 46–50 % of the patients achieved a CR. This trial demonstrated that ondansetron and granisetron are equally effective at preventing acute nausea and vomiting associated with conditioning regimens frequently used prior to HSCT. Overall, although cross-comparison of studies is hindered by too many different variables, the results of a two-drug combination of a first-generation 5-HT$_3$ receptor antagonist and dexamethasone are less impressive for high-dose chemotherapy than those for conventional-dose highly emetogenic chemotherapy. Clearly, new agents and approaches are needed.

8.4 Palonosetron for High-Dose Multiple-Day Chemotherapy

The unique pharmacology of palonosetron, a second-generation 5-HT$_3$ receptor antagonist, is thought to partly explain its improved efficacy against delayed CINV [26–28]. Palonosetron has not only greater 5-HT$_3$ receptor binding affinity and longer plasma elimination half-life compared with older antagonists but also a unique interaction with the 5-HT$_3$ receptor at the molecular level. It has been provided evidence that palonosetron exhibits allosteric interactions and positive cooperativity with the 5-HT$_3$ receptor and that these characteristics are not displayed by ondansetron and granisetron [29]. The binding of palonosetron elicits receptor internalization which results in a prolonged inhibition of serotonin signaling [30]. Finally, palonosetron inhibits cross-talk between 5-HT$_3$ and NK-1 signaling pathways [31]. Overall, these properties of palonosetron could offer advantages of both efficacy and convenience over older antagonists as the drug may continue to maintain effective 5-HT$_3$ receptor blockade even when it is no longer detectable in plasma.

In a meeting abstract, Marcacci et al. reported the results of a single-center prospective trial that evaluated the efficacy of palonosetron in patients undergoing high-dose chemotherapy prior to auto-HSCT for a variety of hematological and solid malignancies [32]. A total of 60 patients were accrued in two sequential cohorts ($n=30$ for each) of antiemetic coverage. In the first cohort, patients received a single intravenous dose of palonosetron (0.25 mg) in combination with dexamethasone (8 mg) before chemotherapy initiation, while in the second cohort, a further dose of both palonosetron and dexamethasone was administered on day 3 following chemotherapy initiation. The most common chemotherapy regimen was high-dose melphalan used in 47 % of the patients, followed by BEAM in 42 % of the patients. The study end points were the rates of CR (defined as no emesis and no rescue antiemetics) in the acute (day 1) and delayed (days 2–5 after chemotherapy initiation), while the impact of CINV on daily activities was assessed by the FLIE questionnaire. No differences were observed between the two treatment cohorts in the rate of acute CR (98 % for each). Among the patients who received two doses of palonosetron, there was a trend for a better control of delayed nausea compared with those in the single-dose cohort (delayed nausea: 53 % vs. 77 %; $P=0.06$). In addition, the median value of FLIE nausea score was significantly higher in patients receiving two doses of palonosetron compared with those in the single-dose cohort (55.3 vs. 40.9, respectively; $P=0.0009$). These preliminary results indicated that double dosing of palonosetron and dexamethasone, either given on days 1 and 3 after chemotherapy initiation, may achieve a high control of both acute and delayed CINV and significantly reduce the impact of nausea on daily activities in patients undergoing high-dose multiple-day chemotherapy.

The main results of fully published studies assessing the efficacy of palonosetron in patients undergoing high-dose multiple-day chemotherapy are summarized in Table 8.1. Overall, limited data are currently available to judge the efficacy of palonosetron in this challenging setting. However, in the published studies, palonosetron was shown to have good efficacy and high tolerability, when used in combination with dexamethasone. Current available evidence also suggests that the use of palonosetron in this setting may offer potential efficacy advantages over older 5-HT$_3$ receptor antagonists.

Table 8.1 Summary of fully published studies investigating the efficacy of palonosetron in patients undergoing high-dose multiple-day chemotherapy

Study (number of patients)	Chemotherapy regimen	Antiemetic prophylaxis (dose in mg)	Primary study end point[a]	Overall results
Rzepecki et al. [33] (N=23)	BEAM CARBOPEC BuCY	Palo (0.25) i.v. on day 1 Dex (20) i.v. on day 1, then Dex (12) i.v. daily during chemotherapy	Highly plus moderately effective responses	*Acute phase*: BEAM 70 % CARBOPEC 15 % BuCY 32 % *Delayed phase*: BEAM 100 % CARBOPEC 25 % BuCY 60 %
Ripaldi et al. [34] (N=43 children)	TBI/TY/CY TBI/Ara-C Bu/CY/LPAM BU/LPAM Other	Palo (0.005/kg) i.v. on day 1	Complete control	68 %
Mattiuzzi et al. [35] (N=143)	Flu/ara-C Ida/ara-C	*Arm 1*: Onda (8) bolus + (24) c.i. on each day of chemotherapy *Arm 2*: Palo (0.25) i.v. on each day of ara-C treatment *Arm 3*: Palo (0.25) i.v. on days 1, 3, and 5 of ara-C treatment	Complete response	*Arm 1*: 21 % *Arm 2*: 31 % *Arm 3*: 35 % (P=0.32)
Musso et al. [36] (N=82)	BEAM FEAM Ida/Ara-C	Palo (0.25) i.v. on day 1 Dex (8) i.v. on day 1, then Dex (8) i.v. every other day during chemotherapy	Complete response	46 %

(continued)

Table 8.1 (continued)

Study (number of patients)	Chemotherapy regimen	Antiemetic prophylaxis (dose in mg)	Primary study end point[a]	Overall results
Giralt et al. [37] (*N*=73)	HD melphalan	*Arm 1*: Palo (0.25) i.v. on day 1 *Arm 2*: Palo (0.25) i.v. on days 1 and 2 *Arm 3*: Palo (0.25) i.v. on days 1, 2, and 3 Dex (20) i.v. to all patients on days 1 and 2	Complete protection	*Arm 1*: 42 % *Arm 2*: 42 % *Arm 3*: 44 % (*P*=0.43)
Mirabile et al. [38] (*N*=58)	Ara-C based[b] Mel based[c] Other	Palo (0.25) i.v. on day 1, then every other day until chemotherapy completion Dex (16) i.v. daily during chemotherapy	Complete control	81 %
Yeh et al. [39] (*N*=27)	Flu/Bu TBI/CY RIC	Palo (0.25) i.v. on day 1, then every other day until chemotherapy completion Dex (10–15) i.v. daily during chemotherapy	No vomiting, no nausea	*Conditioning*: no vomiting: 37 %; no nausea: 22 % *Posttransplant*: no vomiting: 37 %; no nausea: 11 %
Chou et al. [40] (*N*=28)	TBI/Flu/CY TBI/CY Bu/CY HD melphalan BEAM	Palo (0.25) i.v. 12 h prior to conditioning, then every 60 h until chemotherapy completion Dex (10) i.v. daily during chemotherapy	No vomiting, no nausea	*Acute phase*: no vomiting: 29 %; no nausea: 11 % *Delayed phase*: no vomiting: 61 % No nausea: 11 %

Palo palonosetron, *Dex* dexamethasone, *BEAM* BCNU/etoposide/ara-C/melphalan, *CARBOPEC* carboplatin/etoposide/cyclophosphamide, *Bu* busulfan, *CY* cyclophosphamide, *TBI* total body irradiation, *TY* thiotepa, *LPAM* melphalan, *Flu* fludarabine, *Ida* idarubicin, *FEAM* fotemustine/etoposide/ara-C/melphalan, *RIC* reduced-intensity conditioning

[a]See text for more details

[b]Regimens containing cytarabine at a dose of 4 g/m^2 per day

[c]Regimens containing melphalan at a single dose of 140–180 mg/m^2

A single-center study evaluated the efficacy of palonosetron plus dexamethasone in preventing both acute and delayed emesis following conditioning prior to HSCT using a historical cohort of patients (*n*=23) treated with ondansetron as a control [33]. Among the 46 evaluated patients, 20 of them received BEAM chemotherapy for malignant lymphoma, 16 patients were treated with carboplatin/etoposide/cyclophosphamide (CARBOPEC) for a relapsed germ-cell tumor, and the remaining 10 patients received Bu/CY chemotherapy for acute myeloid leukemia.

Antiemetic outcome was assessed as highly effective response (defined as either no emesis and no more than moderate nausea or one to two emetic episodes and no more than mild nausea) and moderately effective response (defined as no emesis but severe nausea or one to two emetic episodes and moderate nausea or three to four emetic episodes and no more than mild nausea). The acute study period started with chemotherapy initiation and continued for 24 h after therapy completion, while the delayed study period was 5 days after chemotherapy completion. The efficacy results suggested that a single-dose palonosetron plus a daily dosing of dexamethasone is significantly superior to a daily dosing of ondansetron and dexamethasone for the prevention of both acute (highly plus moderately effective responses: 70 % vs. 35 % for BEAM, 15 % vs. 5 % for CARBOPEC, and 32 % vs. 20 % for Bu/CY) and delayed (100 % vs. 50 % for BEAM, 25 % vs.10 % for CARBOPEC, and 60 % vs. 30 % for Bu/CY) CINV in patients undergoing conditioning chemotherapy prior to HSCT.

Ripaldi et al. reported the results of a retrospective review that evaluated the efficacy of palonosetron alone to control nausea and vomiting in a cohort of 43 children undergoing conditioning prior to HSCT [34]. Median age at transplantation was 10 years. The majority of patients suffered from acute leukemia (51 %). A total of 47 transplantation procedures were carried out, of which 26 were allogeneic and 21 were autologous. Antiemetic efficacy was assessed as CC, defined as ≤ 1 emetic episode per day, and no nausea. Delayed vomiting that occurred more than 10 days after the start of conditioning was excluded from analysis. The authors concluded that palonosetron is a valuable option for the prevention of chemotherapy and radiotherapy-induced nausea and vomiting in children undergoing HSCT.

In a randomized prospective trial, two extended schedules of palonosetron (0.25 mg/day) from day 1 to day 5 or on days 1, 3, and 5 were compared with daily ondansetron in 143 patients suffering from acute myeloid leukemia or high-risk myelodysplastic syndrome who received induction chemotherapy or first salvage regimen with high-dose (greater than 1.5 g/m^2 up to 5 days) cytarabine-containing regimens [35]. Patients were followed for a total of 7 days, starting with the first day of chemotherapy. The primary end point of the study was the rate of CR (defined as no emesis and no use of rescue antiemetics) during the 7-day study period. Although more patients in each palonosetron arm than in the ondansetron arm achieved CR, this difference was not statistically significant ($P=0.32$). The results of this study with a limited number of patients also showed that significantly more patients in the palonosetron on days 1–5 arm than in the ondansetron arm and in the palonosetron on days 1, 3, and 5 arm experienced no or mild delayed nausea on days 6 (95 % vs. 73 % vs. 72 %, respectively; $P=0.001$) and 7 (98 % vs. 80 % vs. 86 %; $P=0.02$). The most common treatment-related adverse events were constipation and headache. The investigators concluded that palonosetron given daily for 4 or 5 days significantly reduces the incidence and severity of nausea on days 6 and 7 in patients receiving multiple-day chemotherapy with a high-dose cytarabine-containing regimen.

A single-center prospective trial evaluated a single dose of palonosetron in combination with daily dosing of dexamethasone for the prevention of CINV in 134 patients undergoing either single-day ($n=52$) or multiple-day ($n=82$) high-dose chemotherapy as conditioning prior to auto-HSCT for hematological malignancies [36]. The primary end point of the study was the rate of CR (defined as no emesis and no rescue antiemetics) during the conditioning regimen and within 5 days after the end of chemotherapy. The study results were encouraging, but a subgroup analysis showed differences in efficacy among the different conditioning regimens (CR: 38 % for BEAM/FEAM and 74 % for idarubicin/ara-C). It also should be noted that a large number of patients who received a second dose of palonosetron for breakthrough emesis were successfully rescued.

A randomized, double-blind pilot study explored the efficacy and safety of palonosetron for the prevention of CINV in multiple-myeloma patients receiving high-dose melphalan for 2 days prior to HSCT [37]. Patients were assigned to one of three cohorts receiving palonosetron for 1, 2, or 3 days. The primary study end point was the rate of complete protection (CP), defined as no emesis throughout the cumulative 7-day study period. This pilot study with a limited number of patient showed that the 1-, 2-, or 3-day palonosetron dosing cohorts were not statistically different from each other ($P=0.43$). Most adverse events were of mild-to-moderate intensity and, in the investigator's opinion, unrelated to study medication. However, daily dosing of palonosetron is likely to have little to no advantage over an every-other-day schedule due to the pharmacology of the antagonist. More recently, patients suffering from different hematological and solid malignancies were enrolled in a single-center prospective trial to explore the efficacy of an every-other-day palonosetron schedule for the prevention of CINV caused by a variety of high-dose multiple-day chemotherapy regimens [38]. The primary efficacy end point of the study was the rate of CC (defined as no emesis, no rescue antiemetics, and no more than mild nausea) during the overall study period. The overall period started with the initiation of chemotherapy (day 1) and continued for 24 h after the last dose of chemotherapy (overall study period). Historical control patients received an intravenous ondansetron dose of 16 mg per day in combination with the same daily dose of dexamethasone (16 mg), both administered on each day of chemotherapy duration. The average number of days of chemotherapy was 4.7 days (range, 2–6 days) and 4.3 days (range, 2–6 days) in the palonosetron and historical cohorts, respectively. Significantly, more patients in the palonosetron cohort had undergone auto-HSCT as part of frontline therapy compared with those in the historical cohort (46 % vs. 20 %, respectively; $P=0.003$). The proportion of patients achieving CC in the palonosetron cohort was significantly higher than that observed in the ondansetron cohort during the overall study period (81 % vs. 50 %, respectively; $P=0.001$). In a multivariable analysis, both the use of palonosetron ($P=0.001$) and a longer duration of chemotherapy ($P=0.01$) independently predicted a better outcome to antiemetic treatment.

In a small-size prospective trial, the efficacy of an every-other-day palonosetron schedule combined with daily dexamethasone dosing was evaluated during the entire conditioning period prior to allo-HSCT in patients with hematological disorders [39]. The majority of patients (63 %) received a myeloablative conditioning regimen. The control of nausea and vomiting was assessed on a daily basis from the start of conditioning to day 7 after HSCT. The authors concluded that palonosetron every other day combined with dexamethasone is effective in preventing emesis during conditioning, but nausea is less effectively prevented, especially in the first week after HSCT.

At a single center, consecutive patients undergoing a variety of conditioning regimens, with or without TBI, prior to allo-HSCT for various hematological diseases were retrospectively reviewed [40]. Patients who received either daily dosing of a first-generation 5-HT$_3$ receptor antagonist or palonosetron administered every 60 h during the conditioning were stratified into the standard ($n=23$) and palonosetron ($n=28$) groups, respectively. Daily intravenous dexamethasone was also administered to all patients. Acute emesis was defined as nausea or vomiting occurring during and 24 h after conditioning, whereas delayed emesis was defined as nausea or vomiting occurring between 24 and 120 h after completing the conditioning regimen. In this retrospective review with a limited number of patients, palonosetron and older antagonists were at least equally effective for the control of emesis in allo-HSCT recipients. However, the majority of patients (52 %) in the standard group required rescue antiemetics, compared with only 21 % of the patients in the palonosetron group ($P=0.04$).

8.5 NK-1 Receptor Antagonists for High-Dose Multiple-Day Chemotherapy

Aprepitant was the first NK-1 receptor antagonist introduced into clinical care. When used for 3 days as approved by the FDA, aprepitant improves the antiemetic efficacy of 5-HT$_3$ receptor antagonists and dexamethasone, particularly in the setting of delayed emesis [41, 42]. Conditioning regimens prior to HSCT typically take up to a week to administer, and therefore aprepitant should be continued longer than the drug is currently used. In addition, aprepitant has a complex metabolic pathway because it is both a substrate and moderate inhibitor of the cytochrome-P450 3A4 system, which could lead to clinically significant toxicity implications [43]. Since both etoposide and cyclophosphamide are metabolized by this enzyme, aprepitant could theoretically affect the transplantation outcome as well as regimen-related toxicity. However, two recent reports did not show significant drug interaction of aprepitant with cyclophosphamide as well as negative effects on melphalan pharmacokinetics in cancer patients undergoing conditioning prior to HSCT [44, 45]. The main results of fully published studies assessing the efficacy of aprepitant in patients undergoing high-dose multiple-day chemotherapy are summarized in Table 8.2. Interpretation of the data from most studies is hindered by several factors, including the small sample size, variable antiemetic dosing regimens, and nonuniformity of the efficacy end points.

In a pilot trial, the efficacy of an antiemetic regimen containing aprepitant was evaluated for the prevention of CINV caused by conditioning regimens prior to

Table 8.2 Summary of fully published studies investigating the efficacy of aprepitant in patients undergoing high-dose multiple-day chemotherapy

Study (number of patients)	Chemotherapy regimen	Antiemetic prophylaxis (dose in mg)	Primary study end point[a]	Overall results
Paul et al. [46] (N=42)	BEAM HD melphalan Bu/CY Other	Onda (24) or Dola (100) p.o. on day 1 Dex (12) p.o. on day 1 Apr (125) p.o. on day 1, then Apr (80) p.o. daily during chemotherapy	Complete emetic response	54 %
Jordan et al. [47] (N=64)	T/ICE HD melphalan	Gra (1) i.v. on each day of chemotherapy Dex (8) i.v. daily until 2 days after chemotherapy Apr (125) p.o. on day 1, then Apr (80) daily until 2 days after chemotherapy	Complete response	63 %
Pielichowski et al. [48] (N=56)	BEAM	Palo (0.25) i.v. on day 1 Dex (20) i.v. on day 1, then Dex (12) i.v. on each day of chemotherapy Apr (125) p.o. on day 1, then Apr (80) p.o. on days 2 and 3	Highly effective response	*Overall phase*: 82 % *Acute phase*: 94 % *Delayed phase*: 85 %
Pielichowski et al. [49] (N=20)	Bu/CY	Palo (0.25) i.v. on day 1 Dex (20) i.v. on day 1, then Dex (12) i.v. on each day of chemotherapy Apr (125) p.o. on day 1, then Apr (80) p.o. on days 2 and 3	Highly effective response	*Overall phase*: 55 % *Acute phase*: 70 % *Delayed phase*: 55 %
Uchida et al. [50] (N=26)	MCEC HD melphalan LEED Other	Gra (3) i.v. BID on each day of chemotherapy Apr (125) p.o. on day 1, then Apr (80) p.o. daily during chemotherapy	Complete response	42 %
Uchida et al. [51] (N=46)	TBI/CY Bu/CY Flu/Bu/TBI Flu/CY Flu/Mel/TBI	Gra (3) i.v. BID on each day of chemotherapy and/or TBI Apr (125) p.o. on day 1, then Apr (80) p.o. daily during chemotherapy	Complete response	48 %

Table 8.2 (continued)

Stiff et al. [52] (N=179)	TBI/CY Bu/CY TBI/VP/CY BCV	*Arm 1*: Onda (8) p.o. TID on day 1, then every day until 1 day after chemotherapy	Complete response	*Arm 1*: 82 % *Arm 2*: 66 % (*P*<0.001)
		Dex (7.5) i.v. daily until 1 day after chemotherapy		
		Apr (125) p.o. on day 1, then Apr (80) p.o. daily until 3 days after chemotherapy		
		Arm 2: Onda (8) p.o. TID on day 1, then every day until 1 day after chemotherapy		
		Dex (10) i.v. daily until 1 day after chemotherapy		
		Placebo p.o. daily until 3 days after chemotherapy		
Deauna-Limayo et al. [53] (N=18)	BEAM HD melphalan	Palo (0.25) i.v. daily during chemotherapy, then Palo (0.25) i.v. on day 3 after transplant	Complete control	*Acute phase*: 78 % *Delayed phase*: 33 % *Overall phase*: 17 %
		Dex (4) i.v. daily during chemotherapy		
		Apr (125) p.o. on day 1, then Apr (80) p.o. on days 2 and 3		
Sakurai et al. [54] (N=20)	Flu/Mel with or without TBI	Onda (4) i.v. BID during the 2 days of melphalan	Complete response	35 %
		Methylprednisolone (62.5) i.v. BID during the 2 days of melphalan		
		Apr (125) p.o. starting 1 day after the second dose of melphalan, then Apr (80) p.o. daily for 4 days		

Palo palonosetron, *Dex* dexamethasone, *Onda* ondansetron, *Dola* dolasetron, *Gra* granisetron, *Apr* aprepitant, *BID* twice daily, *TID* three times a day, *BEAM* BCNU/etoposide/ara-C/melphalan, *Bu* busulfan, *CY* cyclophosphamide, *T/ICE* paclitaxel/ifosfamide/carboplatin/etoposide, *MCEC* ranimustine/carboplatin/etoposide/cyclophosphamide, *LEED* etoposide/cyclophosphamide/melphalan/dexamethasone, *TBI* total body irradiation, *Flu* fludarabine, *VP* etoposide, *BCV* BCNU/cyclophosphamide/VP16, *Mel* melphalan
[a]See text for more details

HSCT [46]. The majority of patients had a primary cancer diagnosis of multiple myeloma or malignant lymphoma. Eight different chemotherapeutic regimens with varying duration and emetogenic potential including TBI were used in the study. The primary end point was the rate of complete emetic response (CER; defined as no episodes of emesis, none-to-mild nausea, and no rescue antiemetics) that was evaluated daily beginning on day 1 and continuing up to day 7 following chemotherapy. In this exploratory trial, addition of aprepitant to the 1-day regimen of a

5-HT$_3$ receptor antagonist plus dexamethasone failed to meet the primary objective of increasing CER rates by 20 % on each of the 7 days after chemotherapy initiation.

Jordan et al. prospectively evaluated the triple combination of aprepitant, granisetron, and dexamethasone in patients undergoing conditioning regimens prior to auto-HSCT for either multiple myeloma or a solid tumor [47]. The primary end point was the rate of CR (defined as no vomiting and no rescue antiemetics) in the overall study period (day 1 until 5 days after chemotherapy completion). For the acute phase (i.e., during days of chemotherapy administration), a CR was achieved in 53 patients (83 %), while 45 patients (70 %) experienced delayed CR during the period of 5 days after chemotherapy completion. The tolerability of the aprepitant regimen over 4–5 days was comparable with the 3-day dose regimen. The authors concluded that the addition of aprepitant to the standard antiemetic regimen may afford improved control of CINV during high-dose multiple-day chemotherapy administration.

A single-center study was performed to assess a triple-drug combination of aprepitant, palonosetron, and dexamethasone in the prevention of both acute and delayed emesis caused by BEAM chemotherapy prior to auto-HSCT for malignant lymphoma [48]. The study included historical control patients who received ondansetron (32 mg intravenously daily during chemotherapy; $n = 20$) or single-dose palonosetron ($n = 20$), either in combination with daily dexamethasone. Antiemetic outcome was assessed as highly effective response (defined as either no emesis and no more than moderate nausea or one to two emetic episodes and no more than mild nausea) in the acute (day 1 until 24 h after chemotherapy completion) and delayed (5 days after chemotherapy completion) study periods. This small-size study with historical control cohorts showed that the addition of aprepitant to palonosetron and dexamethasone is significantly superior to palonosetron or ondansetron, both with dexamethasone, for the prevention of both acute (highly effective response: 94 % vs. 70 % vs. 35 %, respectively) and delayed (85 % vs. 85 % vs. 50 %) CINV in patients undergoing BEAM chemotherapy with HSCT. Another similar study with historical control patients was carried out from the same group to evaluate the efficacy of the triple-drug combination in preventing both acute and delayed emesis caused by Bu/CY chemotherapy as conditioning prior to allo-HSCT for hematological malignancies [49]. The patients treated with the triple-drug combination had significantly higher response rates than those receiving palonosetron ($n = 20$) or ondansetron ($n = 20$), both with dexamethasone, during both the acute (highly effective response: 70 % vs. 30 % vs. 20 %, respectively) and delayed (55 % vs. 55 % vs. 30 %) study periods.

Uchida et al. retrospectively evaluated the effectiveness and safety of aprepitant in addition to granisetron in Japanese patients with hematological malignancies receiving conditioning prior to auto-HSCT [50]. There was a historical cohort of 22 patients receiving granisetron alone as a control. Since most patients in the study were already highly immunosuppressed, corticosteroids were not administered for emetic control. Aprepitant was administered for up to 6 days depending on each individual conditioning regimen (range, 3–6 days). The primary end point was the rate of CR (defined as no emesis with only grade 1–2 nausea, using the Common Terminology Criteria for Adverse Events v.4) during chemotherapy and until 5 days after the last dose was administered. The proportion of patients who achieved a CR in the aprepitant group was significantly higher than that in the control group (42 % vs. 5 %, respectively; $P=0.003$). The frequencies of drug-related adverse events were not significantly different between two treatment groups. In addition, the same authors retrospectively assessed the efficacy and safety of aprepitant added to granisetron in the setting of high-dose chemotherapy with allo-HSCT for hematological malignancies [51]. The control cohort included 42 consecutive patients who received granisetron alone. The rate of CR in the aprepitant group was significantly higher than that in the control group (48 % vs. 24 %, respectively; $P=0.02$). Overall, the findings from these two retrospective reviews suggested that the addition of aprepitant to granisetron can improve the antiemetic efficacy without influencing toxicities in patients undergoing high-dose chemotherapy prior to either autologous or allogeneic HSCT.

Recently, Stiff et al. performed a randomized, placebo-controlled, phase III trial of aprepitant in combination with ondansetron and dexamethasone in patients treated with myeloablative regimens before autologous or allogeneic HSCT [52]. Eligible patients who had hematological malignancies were randomized to receive oral aprepitant or placebo daily during and for 3 days after chemotherapy completion. The primary efficacy end point of the study was the rate of CR (defined as no emesis and none-to-mild nausea) during the entire period of aprepitant administration. Secondary efficacy end points included number of emetic episodes, severity of nausea assessed using a 100-mm visual analog scale (VAS), need for rescue antiemetics, and transplantation outcome, including regimen-related toxicity (RRT). For the primary and secondary end points, the data were analyzed as composite responses (average daily responses) to account for the different lengths of the conditioning regimens, which ranged from 5 to 8 days. The RRT was also measured by documenting engraftment and all non-myelosuppressive grade 3 or 4 toxicity during and after the first 30 days after the last dose of aprepitant. The study was powered to show a 20 % difference between the antiemetic regimens. The rate of CR in the aprepitant group was significantly higher than that in the placebo group ($P<0.001$). Proportions of patients with no emesis all days were 73 % for the aprepitant group and 22 % for the placebo group ($P<0.001$). There were no between-group differences in the mean VAS scores, amount of rescue antiemetics used, RRT, engraftment, or transplantation outcome. The authors concluded that the addition of aprepitant significantly decreased emesis and significant nausea, whereas had no impact on use of rescue medication, or overall VAS nausea scores.

A pilot study was performed to assess emetic responses to a multiday regimen of palonosetron, aprepitant, and low-dose dexamethasone that was used during consecutive days of conditioning prior to auto-HSCT [53]. An additional single dose of palonosetron was given on day 3 after transplantation. A total of 20 patients with multiple myeloma and malignant lymphoma were enrolled and 18 analyzed. The primary end point of the study was to assess the rate of CC (defined as no emetic episode in each 24-h interval, no rescue antiemetics, and Nausea Visual

Score of ≤2.5) in the acute (24 h following chemotherapy initiation), delayed (day 2 of chemotherapy and up to 72 h after chemotherapy completion), and overall study periods. No patient experienced emetic failure in the overall period. However, nausea remained a major problem with 78 % of the patients developing nausea, although the majority of nauseated patients (61 %) had no significant nausea.

A retrospective comparative study evaluated the efficacy of aprepitant in 60 patients who received high-dose melphalan-based conditioning prior to allo-HSCT for hematological malignancies [54]. Twenty of the 60 patients also received aprepitant for 5 days; the remaining 40 patients, who received ondansetron and methylprednisolone as an antiemetic prophylaxis, served as a control. The overall study period was 12 days from the first day of melphalan administration. The rate of CR (defined as no emesis and no rescue antiemetics) was significantly higher in the aprepitant group than in the control group during the overall study period (35 % vs. 10 %; $P<0.05$). Overall, the results from very different studies indicate that aprepitant has a greater impact on vomiting than it has on nausea. In addition, there is a lack of well-designed and powered randomized studies evaluating aprepitant in combination with palonosetron in the setting of high-dose multiple-day chemotherapy.

More recently, Schmitt et al. reported a randomized, placebo-controlled, double-blind, single-center phase III trial to assess the efficacy of aprepitant in addition to a standard regimen in a homogeneous population of patients who were scheduled to undergo the same conditioning prior to auto-HSCT [55]. A total of 362 patients with multiple myeloma were randomly assigned at a one-to-one ratio to receive either aprepitant (125 mg orally on day 1 and 80 mg orally on days 2–4), granisetron (2 mg orally on days 1–4), and dexamethasone (4 mg orally on day 1 and 2 mg orally on days 2 and 3) or matching placebo, granisetron (2 mg orally on days 1–4), and dexamethasone (8 mg orally on day 1 and 4 mg orally on days 2 and 3). To reduce the risk of infection after HSCT, a lower dose of dexamethasone than generally recommended for highly emetogenic regimens was chosen. High-dose melphalan was administered intravenously on days 1 and 2, while HSCT was performed on day 4. The primary end point of the study was the rate of CR (defined as no emesis and no rescue antiemetics) within 120 h of melphalan administration. The study was powered to show a 15 % difference between the antiemetic regimens. In the overall phase, more patients in the aprepitant arm experienced a CR compared with those in the control arm ($P=0.004$; Fig. 8.1). Significantly, more patients in the aprepitant arm did not experience either emesis or significant nausea (VAS >25 mm) over the 5 days compared with the control arm ($P=0.003$ and $P=0.02$, respectively; Fig. 8.1). However, control of overall nausea was less pronounced (85 % vs. 78 %; $P=0.10$). There was also no between-arm difference in the rescue medication use during the entire study period of 7 days after chemotherapy initiation (48 % vs. 40 %; $P=0.16$). More patients in the aprepitant arm, compared with those in the control arm, had an FLIE score indicating no impact on daily life (74 % vs. 59 %, respectively; $P=0.004$). Rates of adverse events did not significantly differ between the two treatment arms during the entire study period. However, influence of the antiemetic regimens on hematological recovery, progression-free survival, or overall survival was

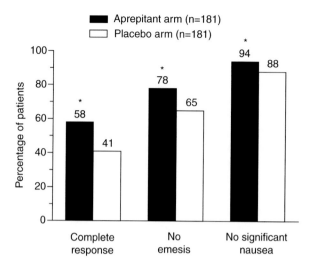

Fig. 8.1 Efficacy of aprepitant in providing complete response (no emesis and no rescue antiemetics), no emesis, and no significant nausea (VAS <25 mm) within 120 h of high-dose melphalan administration. $*P<0.05$ compared with control arm (Data from Schmitt et al. [55])

not assessed in this trial. The authors concluded that the addition of aprepitant to a standard antiemetic regimen should be strongly considered in the setting of high-dose melphalan conditioning.

8.6   Recommendations and Future Directions

High-dose multiple-day chemotherapy remains one of the neglected areas of antiemetic research [56]. There are difficulties in developing evidenced-based recommendations for the optimal strategy of CINV control in this challenging setting [15]. The lack of consistent recommendations and strategies is due to the fact that the larger amount of available information comes from limited series of heterogeneous patient populations, characterized as having a variety of tumor types which have been treated with different chemotherapy regimens administered over consecutive days. Few randomized trials have been done that use different efficacy end points compared to the standard antiemetic trials of conventional-dose chemotherapy. In addition, most patients have experienced emesis with prior chemotherapy or irradiation. It also must be pointed out that both acute and delayed CINV may occur on day 2 or subsequent chemotherapy days, delayed symptoms may occur after chemotherapy completion, and patients often receive narcotic analgesics and/or other medications which may be a risk factor for emesis [2, 47]. The current treatment recommendations for the management of CINV caused by high-dose multiple-day chemotherapy are mainly extrapolated from nonrandomized studies of patients who have been treated with a first-generation 5-HT$_3$ receptor antagonist alone or in combination with corticosteroids [15]. Accordingly, evidence-based guidelines recommend a two-drug combination of a 5-HT$_3$ receptor antagonist and dexamethasone, either administered on each day of the chemotherapy treatment [57, 58]. In spite of a paucity of randomized trials evaluating palonosetron in patients undergoing high-dose multiple-day chemotherapy, available evidence suggests that the daily dosing required with older antagonists may be not needed with palonosetron in this setting [35, 37–40]. Fewer doses of palonosetron seem necessary to achieve at least the same level of protection against CINV in this special population. Further randomized investigations of long-acting palonosetron could also include the novel transdermal formulation of granisetron that has been developed to provide extended release of the drug over 7 days [59].

The updated guidelines from American Society of Clinical Oncology recommend that the addition of an NK-1 receptor antagonist should be strongly considered, although evidence to support its use is limited [58]. More recently, meaningful prospective data have been added to the current literature to support the use of aprepitant, when also administered beyond day 3 of initiating chemotherapy, as an effective and safe approach in the setting of high-dose chemotherapy with HSCT [54, 55]. It is likely that the findings from randomized trials of aprepitant in this setting will be included in the upcoming version of the antiemetic guidelines from Multinational Association of Supportive Care in Cancer. In light of these results, it would be of interest to examine the effects of combining daily aprepitant with every-other-day dosing of palonosetron versus a daily dosing of aprepitant and an older 5-HT$_3$ receptor antagonist in this setting. It also should be noted that fosaprepitant, an intravenous prodrug for aprepitant, as well as novel NK-1 receptor antagonists such as netupitant and rolapitant have been shown to have a high degree of receptor occupancy for a long duration when given as a single dose and appear to be well tolerated [60, 61]. Clinical investigations are needed to determine how these agents affect control of CINV as well as safety and compliance with antiemetic therapy in the challenging setting of high-dose multiple-day chemotherapy. The optimal dose of dexamethasone is also unknown, and, therefore, the minimum effective doses of corticosteroids remain to be fully investigated because of the possible toxicities of prolonged dosing which can be particularly harmful in patients conditioned prior to HSCT. However, clinicians should keep in mind that the literature data suggest that neither 5-HT$_3$ receptor antagonists nor aprepitant has been very effective in controlling nausea that remains frequent in patients undergoing conventional-dose chemotherapy [62]. Since there were similar findings in the recent phase III trials of aprepitant for high-dose chemotherapy, it also remains a need to improve control of nausea in this setting [54, 55]. Given the previously demonstrated efficacy of the atypical antipsychotic olanzapine against either delayed nausea or breakthrough CINV caused by conventional-dose chemotherapy, it would seem reasonable to postulate that its addition to antiemetic coverage may improve control of nausea, particularly on the latter days of chemotherapy and the posttransplantation period [63, 64]. However, the optimal dose *(10 mg/day or lower)* and tolerability of olanzapine with respect to sedation need exploration in this special population in order to minimize the side-effect burden for patients who are already significantly debilitated by their condition [65]. It must be pointed out that the enrollment of a randomized, placebo-controlled, double-blind, multicenter phase III trial comparing olanzapine (days 1–4) to placebo in combination with a 5-HT$_3$ receptor antagonist (day 1), dexamethasone (days 1–4), and either fosaprepitant (day 1) or aprepitant (days 1–3) in patients treated with single-day, highly emetogenic chemotherapy has just been completed (Alliance trial A221301). The primary end point of the study is the proportion of patients with no nausea in the acute, delayed, and overall study periods, while the incidence of potential toxicities related to olanzapine is one of the secondary end points. The results of this large, placebo-controlled, double-blind study, which are expected shortly, will provide clinicians important information on some issues such as the effectiveness of olanzapine combined with a three-drug regimen, particularly in the control of nausea, and the tolerability profile of this agent when used as an antiemetic at the dose of 10 mg per day. At last but not least, the differences in patient populations (i.e., age, gender, disease state, and prior history of CINV) as well as varied high-dose chemotherapy regimens could influence the comparative responses between antiemetic regimens. Therefore, the most appropriate strategy of investigation using standardized end points of effectiveness should be to evaluate one disease state and one chemotherapy regimen [55]. For the implementation of such a strategy, there is also a need to plan adequately powered trials in the context of a collaborative clinical network in order to complete accrual in a reasonable time frame.

References

1. Aschan J (2007) Risk assessment in haematopoietic stem cell transplantation: conditioning. Best Pract Res Clin Haematol 20:295–310
2. Schwartzberg LS, Jacobs P, Matsuoka P et al (2012) The role of second-generation 5-HT$_3$ receptor antagonists in managing chemotherapy-induced nausea and vomiting in haematological malignancies. Crit Rev Oncol Hematol 83:59–70
3. Selle F, Gligorov J, Richard S et al (2015) Intensive chemotherapy as salvage treatment for solid tumors: focus on germ cell cancer. Braz J Med Biol Res 48:13–24
4. Appelbaum FR (2007) Hematopoietic-cell transplantation at 50. N Engl J Med 357:1472–1475
5. Holtik U, Albrecht M, Chemnitz JM et al (2014) Bone marrow versus peripheral blood allogenic haematopoietic stem cell transplantation for haematological malignancies in adults. Cochrane Database Syst Rev. doi:10.1002/14651858.CD010189.pub2
6. Rolling C, Knop S, Bornhauser M (2014) Multiple myeloma. Lancet. doi:10.1016/S0140-673(14)60493-1
7. Hagemeister FB (2002) Treatment of relapsed aggressive lymphomas: regimens with and without high-dose therapy and stem cell rescue. Cancer Chemother Pharmacol 49(Suppl 1):S13–S20
8. Bastos DA, Feldman DR (2014) The role of high-dose chemotherapy in the management of germ cell tumors. Curr Opin Oncol 26:284–293
9. Hesketh PJ (2008) Chemotherapy-induced nausea and vomiting. N Engl J Med 358:2482–2494
10. Perez EA, Tiemeier T, Solberg LA (1999) Antiemetic therapy for high-dose chemotherapy with transplantation: report of a retrospective analysis of a 5-HT$_3$ regimen and literature review. Support Care Cancer 7:413–424

11. Fetting JH, Grochow LB, Folstein MF et al (1982) The course of nausea and vomiting after high-dose cyclophosphamide. Cancer Treat Rep 66:1487–1493

12. Antman K, Eder JP, Elias A et al (1987) High-dose combination alkylating agent preparative regimen with autologous bone marrow support: the Dana-Farber Cancer Institute/Beth Israel Hospital experience. Cancer Treat Rep 71:119–125

13. Trigg ME, Inverso DM (2008) Nausea and vomiting with high-dose chemotherapy and stem cell rescue therapy: a review of antiemetic regimens. Bone Marrow Transplant 42:501–506

14. Spitzer TR, Grunberg SM, Dicato MA (1998) Antiemetic strategies for high-dose chemoradiotherapy-induced nausea and vomiting. Support Care Cancer 6:233–236

15. Einhorn LH, Grunberg SM, Rapoport B et al (2011) Antiemetic therapy for multiple-day chemotherapy and additional topics consisting of rescue antiemetics and high-dose chemotherapy with stem cell transplant: review and consensus statement. Support Care Cancer 19(suppl 1):S1–S4

16. Jimenez JL, Martin-Ballesteros E, Sureda A et al (2006) Chemotherapy-induced nausea and vomiting in acute leukemia and stem cell transplant patients: results of a multicenter, observational study. Haematologica 91:84–91

17. Adel NG, Khan A, Lucarelli C (2006) Use of palonosetron 0.25 mg IV daily and incidence of nausea and vomiting in patients undergoing bone marrow transplantation. In: 2006 ASCO annual meeting proceedings part I. J Clin Oncol 24:664s

18. De Mulder PHM, Roila F, Kris MG et al (1998) Consensus regarding multiple day and rescue antiemetic therapy. Support Care Cancer 6:248–252

19. Stroncek DF, Fautsch SK, Lasky LC et al (1991) Adverse reactions in patients transfused with cryopreserved marrow. Transfusion 31:521–526

20. del Giglio A, Soares HP, Caparroz C et al (2000) Granisetron is equivalent to ondansetron for prophylaxis of chemotherapy-induced nausea and vomiting: results of a meta-analysis of randomized controlled trials. Cancer 89:2301–2308

21. Jordan K, Hinke A, Grothey A et al (2005) Granisetron versus tropisetron for prophylaxis of acute chemotherapy-induced emesis: a pooled analysis. Support Care Cancer 13:26–31

22. Slaby J, Trneny M, Prochazka B et al (2000) Antiemetic efficacy of three serotonin antagonists during high-dose chemotherapy and autologous stem cell transplantation in malignant lymphoma. Neoplasma 47:319–322

23. Fox-Geiman MP, Fisher SG, Kiley K et al (2001) Double-blind comparative trial of oral ondansetron versus oral granisetron versus IV ondansetron in the prevention of nausea and vomiting associated with highly emetogenic preparative regimens prior to stem cell transplantation. Biol Blood Marrow Transplant 7:596–603

24. Matsuoka S, Okamoto S, Watanabe R et al (2003) Granisetron plus dexamethasone versus granisetron alone in the prevention of vomiting induced by conditioning for stem cell transplantation: a prospective randomized study. Int J Hematol 77:86–90

25. Walsh T, Morris AK, Holle LM et al (2004) Granisetron vs ondansetron for the prevention of nausea and vomiting in hematopoietic stem cell transplant patients: results of a prospective, double-blind, randomized trial. Bone Marrow Transplant 34:963–968

26. Aapro MS, Grunberg SM, Manikhas GM et al (2006) A phase III, double-blind, randomized trial of palonosetron compared with ondansetron in preventing chemotherapy-induced nausea and vomiting following highly emetogenic chemotherapy. Ann Oncol 17:1441–1449

27. Saito M, Aogi K, Sekine I et al (2009) Palonosetron plus dexamethasone versus granisetron plus dexamethasone for prevention of nausea and vomiting during chemotherapy: a double-blind, double-dummy, randomized, comparative phase III trial. Lancet Oncol 10:115–124

28. Celio L, Frustaci S, Denaro A et al (2011) Palonosetron in combination with 1-day versus 3-day dexamethasone for prevention of nausea and vomiting following moderately emetogenic chemotherapy: a randomized, multicenter, phase III trial. Support Care Cancer 19:1217–1225

29. Rojas C, Stathis M, Thomas AG et al (2008) Palonosetron exhibits unique molecular interactions with the 5-HT3 receptor. Anesth Analg 107:469–478

30. Rojas C, Thomas AG, Alt J et al (2010) Palonosetron triggers 5-HT(3) receptor internalization and causes prolonged inhibition of receptor function. Eur J Pharmacol 626:193–199

31. Rojas C, Li Y, Zhang J et al (2010) The antiemetic 5-HT3 receptor antagonist palonosetron inhibits substance P-mediated responses in vitro and in vivo. J Pharmacol Exp Ther 335:362–368
32. Marcacci G, Becchimanzi C, Arcamone M et al (2009) Single vs double dose palonosetron for the prevention of acute and delayed nausea and vomiting in patients undergoing high-dose chemotherapy and autologous stem cell transplantation. In: Joint ECCO 15-34th ESMO Mulidisciplinary Congress Berlin, 20–24 September 2009, Abstract Book. Eur J Cancer 7:574
33. Rzepecki P, Pielichowski W, Oborska S et al (2009) Palonosetron in prevention of nausea and vomiting after highly emetogenic chemotherapy before haematopoietic stem cell transplantation – single center experience. Transplant Proc 41:3247–3249
34. Ripaldi M, Parasole R, De Simone G et al (2010) Palonosetron to prevent nausea and vomiting in children undergoing BMT: efficacy and safety. Bone Marrow Transplant 45:1663–1664
35. Mattiuzzi GN, Cortes JE, Blamble DA et al (2010) Daily palonosetron is superior to ondansetron in the prevention of delayed chemotherapy-induced nausea and vomiting in patients with acute myelogenous leukemia. Cancer 116:5659–5666
36. Musso M, Scalone R, Crescimanno A et al (2010) Palonosetron and dexamethasone for prevention of nausea and vomiting in patients receiving high-dose chemotherapy with auto-SCT. Bone Marrow Transplant 45:123–127
37. Giralt SA, Mangan KF, Maziarz RT et al (2011) Three palonosetron regimens to prevent CINV in myeloma patients receiving multiple-day high-dose melphalan and hematopoietic stem cell transplantation. Ann Oncol 22:939–946
38. Mirabile A, Celio L, Magni M et al (2014) Evaluation of an every-other-day palonosetron schedule to control emesis in multiple-day high-dose chemotherapy. Future Oncol 10:2569–2578
39. Yeh SP, Lo WC, Hsieh CY et al (2014) Palonosetron and dexamethasone for the prevention of nausea and vomiting in patients receiving allogeneic hematopoietic stem cell transplantation. Support Care Cancer 22:1199–1206
40. Chou CW, Chen YK, Yu YB et al (2014) Palonosetron versus first-generation 5-hydroxytryptamine type 3 receptor antagonists for emesis prophylaxis in patients undergoing allogeneic hematopoietic stem cell transplantation. Ann Hematol 93:1225–1232
41. Hesketh PJ, Grunberg SM, Gralla RJ et al (2003) The oral neurokinin-1 antagonist aprepitant for the prevention of chemotherapy-induced nausea and vomiting: a multinational, randomized, double-blind, placebo-controlled trial in patients receiving high-dose cisplatin – The Aprepitant Protocol 052 Study Group. J Clin Oncol 21:4112–4119
42. Schmoll HJ, Aapro MS, Poli-Bigelli S et al (2006) Comparison of an aprepitant regimen with a multiple-day ondansetron regimen, both with dexamethasone, for antiemetic efficacy in high-dose cisplatin treatment. Ann Oncol 17:1000–1006
43. Aapro MS, Walko CM (2010) Aprepitant: drug-drug interactions in perspective. Ann Oncol 21:2316–2323
44. Bubalo JS, Cherala G, McCune J et al (2012) Aprepitant pharmacokinetics and assessing the impact of aprepitant on cyclophosphamide metabolism in cancer patients undergoing hematopoietic stem cell transplantation. J Clin Pharmacol 52:586–594
45. Egerer G, Eisenlohr K, Gronkowski M et al (2010) The NK$_1$ receptor antagonist aprepitant does not alter the pharmacokinetics of high-dose melphalan chemotherapy in patients with multiple myeloma. Br J Clin Pharmacol 70:903–907
46. Paul B, Trovato JA, Thompson J et al (2010) Efficacy of aprepitant in patients receiving high-dose chemotherapy with hematopoietic stem cell support. J Clin Pharm Pract 16:45–51
47. Jordan K, Jahn F, Jahn P et al (2011) The NK-1 receptor-antagonist aprepitant in high-dose chemotherapy (high-dose melphalan and high-dose T-ICE: paclitaxel, ifosfamide, carboplatin, etoposide): efficacy and safety of a triple antiemetic combination. Bone Marrow Transplant 46:784–789
48. Pielichowski W, Barzal J, Gawronski K et al (2011) A triple-drug combination to prevent nausea and vomiting following BEAM chemotherapy before autologous hematopoietic stem cell transplantation. Transplant Proc 43:3107–3110

49. Pielichowski W, Gawronski K, Mlot B et al (2011) Triple-drug combination in the prevention of nausea and vomiting following busulfan plus cyclophosphamide chemotherapy before allogeneic hematopoietic stem cell transplantation. J Buon 16:541–546

50. Uchida M, Ikesue H, Miyamoto T et al (2013) Effectiveness and safety of antiemetic aprepitant in Japanese patients receiving high-dose chemotherapy prior to autologous hematopoietic stem cell transplantation. Biol Pharm Bull 36:819–824

51. Uchida M, Kato K, Ikesue H et al (2013) Efficacy and safety of aprepitant in allogeneic hematopoietic stem cell transplantation. Pharmacotherapy 33:893–901

52. Stiff PJ, Fox-Geiman MP, Kiley K et al (2013) Prevention of nausea and vomiting associated with stem cell transplant: results of a prospective, randomized trial of aprepitant used with highly emetogenic preparative regimens. Biol Blood Marrow Transplant 19:49–55

53. Deauna-Limayo D, Aljitawi OS, Ganguly S et al (2013) Combined use of multiday palonosetron with aprepitant and low-dose dexamethasone in prevention of nausea and emesis among patients with multiple myeloma and lymphoma undergoing autologous hematopoietic stem cell transplant: a pilot study. J Oncol Pharm Pract 20:263–269

54. Sakurai M, Mori T, Kato J et al (2014) Efficacy of aprepitant in preventing nausea and vomiting due to high-dose melphalan-based conditioning for allogeneic hematopoietic stem cell transplantation. Int J Hematol 99:457–462

55. Schmitt T, Goldschmidt H, Neben K et al (2014) Aprepitant, granisetron, and dexamethasone for prevention of chemotherapy-induced nausea and vomiting after high-dose melphalan in autologous transplantation for multiple myeloma: results of a randomized, placebo-controlled phase III trial. J Clin Oncol 32:3413–3420

56. Olver I, Molassiotis A, Aapro M et al (2011) Antiemetic research: future directions. Support Care Cancer 19(Suppl 1):S49–S55

57. Roila F, Herrstedt J, Aapro M et al (2010) Guideline update for MASCC and ESMO in the prevention of chemotherapy- and radiotherapy-induced nausea and vomiting: results of the Perugia consensus conference. Ann Oncol 21(Suppl 5):v232–v243

58. Basch E, Prestrud AA, Hesketh PJ et al (2011) Antiemetics: American Society of Clinical Oncology clinical practice guideline update. J Clin Oncol 29:4189–4198

59. Boccia RV, Gordan LN, Clark G et al (2011) Efficacy and tolerability of transdermal granisetron for the control of chemotherapy-induced nausea and vomiting associated with moderately and highly multi-day chemotherapy: a randomized, double-blind, phase III study. Support Care Cancer 19:1609–1617

60. Celio L, Ricchini F, De Braud F (2013) Efficacy, safety, and patient acceptability of single-dose fosaprepitant regimen for the prevention of chemotherapy-induced nausea and vomiting. Patient Prefer Adherence 7:391–400

61. Navari RM (2013) Management of chemotherapy-induced nausea and vomiting. Drugs 73:249–262

62. Celio L, Aapro M (2013) Research on chemotherapy-induced nausea: back to the past for an unmeet need? J Clin Oncol 31:1376–1377

63. Navari RM, Gray SE, Kerr AC (2011) Olanzapine versus aprepitant for the prevention of chemotherapy-induced nausea and vomiting: a randomized phase III trial. J Support Oncol 9:188–195

64. Navari RM, Nagy CK, Gray SE (2013) Olanzapine versus metoclopramide for the treatment of breakthrough chemotherapy-induced nausea and vomiting in patients receiving highly emetogenic chemotherapy. Support Care Cancer 21:1655–1663

65. Abe M, Hirashima Y, Kasamatsu Y et al (2015) Efficacy and safety of olanzapine combined with aprepitant, palonosetron, and dexamethasone for preventing nausea and vomiting induced by cisplatin-based chemotherapy in gynecological cancer: KCOG-G1301 phase II trial. Support Care Cancer. doi:10.1007/s00520-015-2829-z

Chapter 9
Clinical Management of CINV

Rudolph M. Navari

9.1 Principles in the Management of CINV

Antiemetic guidelines have been published by NCCN [1], ASCO [2], and MASCC [3]. These guidelines form the basis for the recommendations for the management of CINV. As new information and new studies emerge, the guidelines will evolve to provide the highest quality evidence-based clinical practice.

9.2 Single-Day Chemotherapy

For patients receiving highly emetogenic chemotherapy (HEC), current evidence suggests the following [1–3]:

- Pre-chemotherapy—any of the 5-HT$_3$ receptor antagonists with dexamethasone and one of the available oral neurokinin-1 (NK-1) receptor antagonists. Fosaprepitant may be administered intravenously as an alternative to one of the oral NK-1 receptor antagonists on day 1.

    The guidelines suggest that the combination of cyclophosphamide and doxorubicin should be considered as HEC and the appropriate preventative agents should be used.

- Post-chemotherapy—oral aprepitant on days 2 and 3 (omit if fosaprepitant has been given on day 1) and dexamethasone on days 2–4. No NK-1 receptor antagonist is necessary if the NK-1 receptor antagonist netupitant or rolapitant is given on day 1.

R.M. Navari
Cancer Care Program, Central and South America, World Health Organization,
Indiana University School of Medicine South Bend, South Bend, IN, USA
e-mail: rmnavari@gmail.com

© Springer International Publishing Switzerland 2016
R.M. Navari (ed.), *Management of Chemotherapy-Induced Nausea
and Vomiting: New Agents and New Uses of Current Agents*,
DOI 10.1007/978-3-319-27016-6_9

157

For patients receiving moderately emetogenic chemotherapy (MEC), current evidence suggests the following [1–3]:

- Pre-chemotherapy—the 5-HT$_3$ receptor antagonist palonosetron plus dexamethasone. If palonosetron is not available, ondansetron or granisetron may be employed.
- Post-chemotherapy—dexamethasone on days 2–4.

Antiemetic guidelines of the past [4] have included the available oral first-generation 5-HT$_3$ receptor antagonists as optional therapy for the prevention of delayed emesis, but the level of evidence supporting this practice is low [4–7]. The first-generation 5-HT$_3$ receptor antagonists are no longer recommended for use post-chemotherapy [1–3].

For patients receiving low emetogenic chemotherapy, a single agent in the form of a 5-HT$_3$ receptor antagonist, dexamethasone, or a phenothiazine, depending on the clinical situation, should be used pre-chemotherapy, and an antiemetic following chemotherapy should be given only as needed.

9.3   Treatment of Breakthrough CINV

Breakthrough CINV occurs in patients who develop emesis and/or nausea despite adequate prophylaxis prior to chemotherapy. Phenothiazine, metoclopramide, dexamethasone, or olanzapine may be effective in the treatment of breakthrough nausea and vomiting [3]. A 5-HT$_3$ receptor antagonist may also be effective unless a patient presents with nausea and vomiting that developed following the use of a 5-HT$_3$ receptor antagonist as prophylaxis for chemotherapy- or radiotherapy-induced emesis. It is very unlikely that breakthrough nausea and vomiting will respond to an agent in the same drug class after unsuccessful prophylaxis with an agent with the same mechanism of action.

Patients who develop nausea or vomiting post-chemotherapy (days 1–5) despite adequate prophylaxis should be considered for treatment with a 3-day regimen of oral olanzapine or oral metoclopramide. A recently completed phase III study demonstrated that oral olanzapine (10 mg/day for 3 days) was significantly better than oral metoclopramide (10 mg three times daily for 3 days) in controlling both emesis and nausea in patients receiving HEC who developed breakthrough CINV despite guideline-directed prophylactic antiemetics [8].

It is important to note that the NK-1 receptor antagonists have been approved as additive agent to a 5-HT$_3$ receptor antagonist and dexamethasone for the prevention of CINV. They have not been studied and should not be used to treat breakthrough nausea and vomiting.

9.4   Refractory CINV

Patients who develop CINV during subsequent cycles of chemotherapy despite adequate prophylaxis are considered to have refractory CINV. When antiemetic prophylaxis has not been successful in controlling CINV in earlier cycles, patients should be considered for a change in their prophylactic antiemetic regimen. If anxiety is considered to be a major patient factor in the CINV, a benzodiazepine such as lorazepam or alprazolam can be added to the prophylactic regimen. If the patient is receiving HEC, olanzapine (days 1–3) can be substituted for an NK-1 receptor antagonist in the prophylactic antiemetic regimen [9]. If the patient is receiving MEC, an NK-1 receptor antagonist may be considered to be added the palonosetron and dexamethasone antiemetic regimen [10–12].

9.5 Anticipatory CINV

Anticipatory CINV develops when a patient's CINV is not well controlled in previous chemotherapy cycles, and patients develop nausea and vomiting without any chemotherapy in anticipation of the next chemotherapy cycle. In order to prevent the occurrence of anticipatory CINV, patients should be counseled prior to the initial course of treatment concerning their "expectations" of CINV. Patients should be informed that very effective prophylactic antiemetic regimens will be used and that 70–75 % of patients will have a complete response (no emesis, no use of rescue medications). The most effective prophylactic antiemetic regimen for the patient's specific type of chemotherapy should be used prior to the first course of chemotherapy in order to obtain the optimum control of CINV during the first course of chemotherapy. If CINV is effectively controlled during the first cycle, it is likely that the patient will have effective control during subsequent cycles of the same chemotherapy. If the patient has a poor experience with CINV in the first cycle, it may be more difficult to control CINV in subsequent cycles, and refractory and/or anticipatory CINV may occur. The use of antianxiety medications such as lorazepam or another benzodiazepine may be considered for excess anxiety prior to the first course of chemotherapy in order to obtain an optimum outcome and prevent anticipatory CINV. If anticipatory CINV occurs despite the use of prophylactic antiemetics, behavioral therapy might be considered.

9.6 Multi-day Chemotherapy and High-Dose Chemotherapy with Stem Cell or Bone Marrow Transplantation

Although there have been significant improvements in the prevention of CINV in patients receiving single-day HEC and MEC, there has been limited progress in the prevention of CINV in patients receiving multiple-day chemotherapy or high-dose chemotherapy with stem cell transplant. The current recommendation is to give a first-generation 5-HT$_3$ receptor antagonist and dexamethasone daily during each day of chemotherapy in patients receiving multiple-day chemotherapy or high-dose chemotherapy with stem cell transplant [13]. This regimen appears to be at least partially effective in controlling acute CINV but is not very effective in controlling delayed CINV. The complete response in most studies of 5 days of cisplatin and in various high-dose chemotherapy regimens is 30–70 %, with the majority of studies reporting a complete response of ≤50 % [13].

Patients should receive the appropriate prophylaxis for the emetogenic risk of the chemotherapy for each day of the chemotherapy treatment. Both acute and delayed CINV may occur on day 2 or subsequent chemotherapy days and delayed CINV may occur after the last day of the multi-day chemotherapy treatment.

The antiemetic agents palonosetron, aprepitant, netupitant, rolapitant, and olanzapine have shown effectiveness in controlling both acute and delayed CINV in patients receiving single-day MEC and HEC. They may have application in patients receiving multiple-day or high-dose chemotherapy. Palonosetron has been used in one report of patients receiving 5 days of cisplatin [14], and Albany et al. [15] reported that the addition of aprepitant to a 5-HT$_3$ receptor antagonist and dexamethasone significantly improved the complete response in patients receiving 5 days of cisplatin.

Stiff et al. [16] reported an improvement in nausea and emesis when aprepitant was added to ondansetron and dexamethasone in patients receiving highly emetogenic chemotherapy as a preparative regimen for patients receiving stem cell transplants. Jordan et al. [17] demonstrated some improvement in nausea and emesis when aprepitant was added to granisetron and dexamethasone in patients receiving high-dose chemotherapy (high-dose melphalan and high-dose T-ICE: paclitaxel, ifosfamide, carboplatin, etoposide). Additional studies are needed to define an optimal regimen for the control of CINV in patients receiving preparative chemotherapy regimens for stem cell and bone marrow transplants.

9.7   Prevention and Treatment of Nausea

The current data in the literature from multiple large studies suggest that the first- or second-generation 5-HT$_3$ receptor antagonists and the neurokinin-1 receptor antagonists have not been effective in the control of nausea in patients receiving either MEC or HEC, despite the marked improvement in the control of emesis with these agents [9, 11, 12, 18]. It appears that neither the serotonin nor the substance P receptors may be important in mediating nausea. Recent phase II and phase III studies with olanzapine have demonstrated very good control of both emesis and nausea in patients receiving either MEC or HEC [9, 19, 20]. Preliminary small studies with gabapentin, cannabinoids, and ginger are inconclusive in defining their role, if any, in the prevention of CINV. At this time, olanzapine appears to have high potential for the prevention of both emesis and nausea in patients receiving MEC or HEC [9, 18–20]. If patients are having difficulty with significant nausea, consideration should be given to including olanzapine in their prophylactic antiemetic regimen [9, 18–20]. Olanzapine may also be efficacious in the treatment of breakthrough nausea [8].

References

1. Roila F, Herrstedt J, Aapro M et al (2010) Guideline update for MASCC and ESMO in the prevention of chemotherapy- and radiotherapy-induced nausea and vomiting: results of the Perugia consensus conference. Ann Oncol 21(5):232–243
2. Basch E, Prestrud AA, Hesketh PJ et al (2011) Antiemetic American Society Clinical Oncology clinical practice guideline update. J Clin Oncol 29:4189–4198
3. NCCN Clinical Practice Guidelines in Oncology version 1 2012. Antiemesis. National Comprehensive Cancer Network (NCCN) [online]. Available from URL: http://www.nccn.org/professionals/physician_gls/PDF/antiemesis.pdf. Accessed 30 Sept 2015
4. Kris MG, Hesketh PJ, Somerfield MR et al (2006) American Society of Clinical Oncology guideline for antiemetics in oncology: update 2006. J Clin Oncol 24:2932–2947
5. Navari RM (2003) Pathogenesis-based treatment of chemotherapy-induced nausea and vomiting: two new agents. J Support Oncol 1:89–103
6. Geling O, Eichler H (2005) Should 5-Hydroxytryptamine-3 receptor antagonists be administered beyond 24 hours after chemotherapy to prevent delayed emesis? Systematic re-evaluation of clinical evidence and drug cost implications. J Clin Oncol 23:1289–1294
7. Hickok JT, Roscoe JA, Morrow GR et al (2005) 5-HT$_3$ receptor antagonists versus prochlorperazine for control of delayed nausea caused by doxorubicin: a URCC CCOP randomized controlled trial. Lancet Oncol 6:765–772
8. Navari RM, Nagy CK, Gray SE (2013) Olanzapine versus metoclopramide for the treatment of breakthrough chemotherapy-induced nausea and vomiting in patients receiving highly emetogenic chemotherapy. Support Care Cancer 21:1655–1663
9. Navari RM, Gray SE, Kerr AC (2011) Olanzapine versus aprepitant for the prevention of chemotherapy-induced nausea and vomiting: a randomized phase III trial. J Support Oncol 9:188–195
10. Rapoport BL, Jordon K, Boice JA et al (2010) Aprepitant for the prevention of chemotherapy-induced nausea and vomiting associated with a broad range of moderately emetogenic chemotherapies and tumor types: a randomized, double-blind study. Support Care Cancer 18(4):423–431
11. Navari RM (2015) Profile of netupitant/palonosetron fixed dose combination (NEPA) and its potential in the treatment of chemotherapy-induced nausea and vomiting (CINV). Drug Des Dev Ther 9:155–161
12. Navari RM (2015) Rolapitant for the treatment of chemotherapy induced nausea and vomiting. Expert Rev Anticancer Ther 15:1127–1133
13. Navari RM (2007) Prevention of emesis from multiple-day chemotherapy regimens. J Natl Compr Canc Netw 5:51–59
14. Einhorn LH, Brames ML, Dreicer R et al (2007) Palonosetron plus dexamethasone for the prevention of chemotherapy-induced nausea and vomiting in patients receiving multiple-day cisplatin chemotherapy for germ cell cancer. Support Care Cancer 15:1293–1300
15. Albany C, Brames ML, Fausel C et al (2012) Randomized, double-blind, placebo-controlled, phase III crossover study evaluating the oral neurokinin-1 antagonist aprepitant in combination with a 5-HT$_3$ antagonist plus dexamethasone in patients with germ cell tumor receiving 5-day cisplatin combination chemotherapy regimens: a Hoosier Oncology Group (HOG) study. J Clin Oncol 30:3998–4003
16. Stiff PJ, Fox-German MP, Kiley K et al (2013) Prevention of nausea and vomiting associated with stem cell transplant: results of a prospective, randomized trial of aprepitant used with highly emetogenic preparative regimens. Biol Blood Marrow Transplant 19:49–55
17. Jordan K, Jahn F, Jahn P et al (2011) The NK-1 receptor antagonist aprepitant in high-dose chemotherapy (high dose melphalan and high dose T-ICE: paclitaxel, ifosfamide, carboplatin, etoposide): efficacy and safety of a triple antiemetic combination. Bone Marrow Transpl 46:784–789
18. Navari RM (2012) Treatment of chemotherapy-induced nausea. Community Oncol 9:20–26

19. Navari RM, Einhorn LH, Loehrer PJ et al (2007) A phase II trial of olanzapine, dexametha-
    sone, and palonosetron for the prevention of chemotherapy-induced nausea and vomiting.
    Support Care Cancer 15:1285–1291
20. Tan L, Liu J, Liu X et al (2009) Clinical research of olanzapine for the prevention of
    chemotherapy-induced nausea and vomiting. J Exp Clin Cancer Res 28:1–7

Chapter 10
Treatment of Chemotherapy-Induced Nausea

Rudolph M. Navari

10.1 Introduction

Chemotherapy-induced nausea and vomiting (CINV) is associated with a significant deterioration in quality of life and is perceived by patients as a major adverse effect of the treatment [1]. The use of 5-hydroxytryptamine-3 (5-HT$_3$) receptor antagonists plus dexamethasone has significantly improved the control of CINV [2]. Recent studies have demonstrated additional improvement in the control of CINV with the use of a number of new agents: palonosetron, a second-generation 5-HT$_3$ receptor antagonist [3]; aprepitant, the first agent available in the drug class of neurokinin-1 (NK-1) receptor antagonists [4, 5]; recent introduction of additional NK-1 receptor antagonists netupitant and rolapitant [6, 7]; and olanzapine, an antipsychotic which blocks multiple neurotransmitters in the central nervous system [8–10].

The primary endpoint used for studies evaluating various agents for the control of CINV has been complete response (no emesis, no use of rescue medication) over the acute (24 h post chemotherapy), delayed (24–120 h), and overall (0–120 h) periods [2]. Recent studies have shown that the combination of a 5-HT$_3$ receptor antagonist, dexamethasone, and an NK-1 receptor antagonist has been very effective in controlling emesis in patients receiving either highly emetogenic chemotherapy (HEC) or moderately emetogenic chemotherapy (MEC) over a 120 h period following chemotherapy administration [4–7]. Many of these same studies have measured nausea as a secondary endpoint and have demonstrated that nausea has not been well controlled [2–7].

R.M. Navari, MD, PhD, FACP
Cancer Care Program, Central and South America, World Health Organization,
Atlanta, USA

Student Outreach Clinic, Indiana University School of Medicine South Bend,
South Bend, IN, USA
e-mail: rmnavari@gmail.com

© Springer International Publishing Switzerland 2016   163
R.M. Navari (ed.), *Management of Chemotherapy-Induced Nausea
and Vomiting: New Agents and New Uses of Current Agents*,
DOI 10.1007/978-3-319-27016-6_10

Emesis is a well-defined event which is easily measured, but nausea may be more subjective and more difficult to measure. There are, however, two well-defined measures of nausea which appear to be effective measurement tools which are reproducible: the visual analogue scale (VAS) and the Likert scale [11]. The VAS is a scale from 0 to 10 or 0 to 100 with zero representing no nausea and 10 or 100 representing maximal nausea. The Likert Scale asks patients to rate nausea as none, mild, moderate, or severe.

The purpose of this review is to evaluate the effectiveness of the various antiemetic agents currently in use in the control of chemotherapy-induced nausea and to provide suggestions for the prevention of nausea in the acute, delayed, and overall periods post chemotherapy. Many studies have reported the secondary endpoint of "no significant nausea" or "only mild nausea" [2–7]. This review concentrates on studies that have reported "no nausea" in an attempt to identify the most effective available agents.

10.2 Definition and Pathophysiology

Nausea is a subjective, difficult-to-describe, sick or queasy sensation, usually perceived as being in the stomach that is sometimes followed by emesis [11]. The experience of nausea is difficult to describe in another person because it is a subjective sensation. Nausea and emesis are not necessarily on a continuum. One can experience nausea without emesis and one can have sudden emesis without nausea. Nausea has been assumed to be the conscious awareness of unusual sensations in the "vomiting center" of the brainstem (Fig. 10.1), but the existence of such a center and its relationship to nausea remain controversial [11].

Figure 10.2 illustrates the various receptors that are considered to be involved in CINV.

These receptors are located both in the periphery such as the gastrointestinal tract and in the central nervous system. Various antiemetic agents have been developed as antagonists to the serotonin and the substance-P receptors with relative success in controlling emesis. It is not clear whether the serotonin and/or the substance P receptors are important in the control of nausea. Other receptors such as dopaminergic, histaminic, and muscarinic may be the dominant receptors in the control of nausea [2].

10.3 Antiemetic Agents

10.3.1 First-Generation 5-HT₃ Receptor Antagonists

The 5-HT$_3$ receptor antagonists currently in use include the first-generation serotonin (5-HT$_3$) receptor antagonists dolasetron, granisetron, ondansetron, tropisetron [12], azasetron [13], and ramosetron [14]. These are considered equivalent in efficacy and toxicities when used in the recommended doses, and they have not been

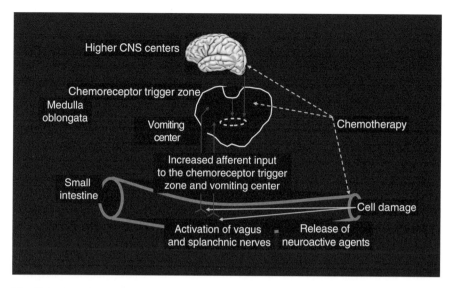

Fig. 10.1 Proposed pathways of chemotherapy-induced emesis and nausea

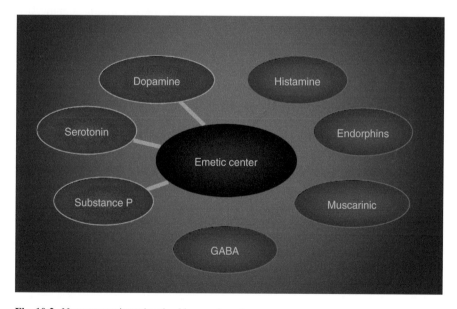

Fig. 10.2 Neurotransmitters involved in emesis and nausea

associated with major toxicities [2]. Azasetron and ramosetron are not available in North American and Europe and have not been compared extensively to the other 5-HT$_3$ receptor antagonists.

In 2006, Canada issued a drug alert for dolasetron, due to the potential of serious cardiovascular adverse events (cardiac arrhythmias) [15], stating that dolasetron was not indicated for use in children but only for prevention of CINV in adults [15]. Subsequently, in 2010, the US Food and Drug Administration (FDA) announced that the intravenous form of dolasetron should no longer be used to prevent CINV in any patient. New data suggested that dolasetron injection can increase the risk of developing a prolongation of the QT interval which may potentially precipitate life-threatening ventricular arrhythmias [16].

The first-generation $5\text{-}HT_3$ receptor antagonists have not been as effective against delayed emesis as they are against acute CINV [17–19]. The first-generation $5\text{-}HT_3$ receptor antagonists alone do not add significant efficacy to that obtained by dexamethasone in the control of delayed emesis [18]. Hickok et al. [19] reported that the first-generation $5\text{-}HT_3$s used in the delayed period were no more effective than prochlorperazine in controlling nausea. The antiemetic effects of prochlorperazine can be attributed to postsynaptic dopamine receptor blockade in the chemoreceptor trigger zone. A meta-analysis [18] showed that there was neither clinical evidence nor considerations of cost-effectiveness to justify using the first-generation $5\text{-}HT_3$ antagonists beyond 24 h after chemotherapy for the prevention of delayed emesis. A number of recent studies have demonstrated that there has been poor control of delayed nausea by the first-generation $5\text{-}HT_3$ receptor antagonists in patients receiving HEC or MEC [10, 20, 21] (Table 10.1). The use of granisetron and dexamethasone in patients receiving highly emetogenic chemotherapy resulted in "no nausea" in 25–27 % of patients [20]. The use of ondansetron plus dexamethasone in patients receiving moderately emetogenic chemotherapy resulted in "no nausea" in 33 % of patients and "no significant nausea" in 56 % of patients [21].

10.3.2   Palonosetron

Palonosetron is a second-generation $5\text{-}HT_3$ receptor antagonist which has antiemetic activity at both central and gastrointestinal sites. In comparison to the first-generation $5\text{-}HT_3$ receptor antagonists, it has a higher potency, a significantly longer half-life, and a different molecular interaction with $5\text{-}HT_3$ receptors [30, 31].

Animal studies have demonstrated that chemotherapy agents produce nausea and vomiting by releasing substance P in the central nervous system and serotonin from the enterochromaffin cells of the small intestine. The released serotonin activates the $5\text{-}HT_3$ receptors located on the vagal afferents to initiate the vomiting reflex. Palonosetron demonstrated a $5\text{-}HT_3$ receptor-binding affinity at least 30-fold higher than other $5\text{-}HT_3$ receptor antagonists [22]. Rojas et al. [31] recently reported that palonosetron exhibited allosteric binding and positive cooperativity when binding to the $5\text{-}HT_3$ receptor compared to simple bimolecular binding for both granisetron and ondansetron. Additional studies by Rojas et al. [31] suggested that palonosetron triggers $5\text{-}HT_3$ receptor internalization and causes prolonged inhibition of receptor function. Differences in binding and effects on receptor function may explain some differences between palonosetron and the first-generation $5\text{-}HT_3$ receptor antago-

Table 10.1 Phase II and III trials of various agents for the treatment of chemotherapy-induced nausea

Study	Chemotherapy	Phase II or III	No. patients	No nausea, delayed (%)		No nausea, overall (%)	
Saito et al. [20]	HEC	III	1114	Palo+Dex:	38*	Palo+Dex:	32*
				Gran+Dex:	27	Gran+Dex:	25
Hesketh et al. [22]	HEC	III	1043			Women:	
						Aprepitant:	46
						Control:	38
						Men:	
						Aprepitant:	50
						Control:	44
Warr et al. [23]				Aprepitant	52*	Aprepitant	48*
				Control	44	Control	42
Warr et al. [21]	Cyclo+Doxo/Epi	III	866	Aprepitant:	37	Aprepitant:	33
				Control:	36	Control:	33
Grote et al. [24]	MEC	II	58	APD:	31	APD:	30
Celio et al. [25]	MEC	III	334	Palo+Dex1:	57	Palo+Dex1:	52
				Palo+Dex3:	62	Palo+Dex3:	57
Aapro et al. [39]	Cyclo+Doxo/Epi	III	300	Palo+Dex1:	50	Palo+Dex1:	47
				Palo+Dex3:	55	Palo+Dex3:	50
Navari et al. [9]	MEC	II	32	OPD:	78	OPD:	78
Tan et al. [10]	MEC	III	229	OAD:	83*	OAD:	83*
				AD:	58	AD:	56
	HEC	III		OAD:	70*	OAD:	70*
				AD:	30	AD:	28
Navari et al. [27]	HEC	III	257	OPD:	69*	OPD:	69*
				APD:	38	APD:	38
Cruz et al. [28]	HEC	III	80	Gabapentin:	72	Gabapentin:	62
				Control:	52	Control:	45
Meiri et al. [29]	MEC, HEC	III	61	No difference between dronabinol or ondansetron		Not reported	
Navari [7]	HEC	III	1070	Rolapitant	56*	Rolapitant	52*
				Control	44	Control	42

Palo palonosetron, *Dex* dexamethasone, *Gran* granisetron, *APD* aprepitant, palonosetron, dexamethasone, *OPD* olanzapine, palonosetron, dexamethasone, *OAD* olanzapine, azasetron, dexamethasone
*$p < 0.05$

nists [3]. These differences may explain palonosetron's efficacy in delayed CINV compared to the first-generation receptor antagonists [3]. A high level of efficacy and an excellent safety profile has been demonstrated in a number of studies [3, 20, 26, 30, 32, 33]. In subgroup analyses in single-dose trials, palonosetron appeared to control nausea better than dolasetron [32] and ondansetron [33] in patients receiving moderately emetogenic chemotherapy.

International antiemetic guidelines suggest the use of a 5-HT$_3$ receptor antagonist and dexamethasone prechemotherapy and dexamethasone post chemotherapy for patients receiving MEC and the use of a 5-HT$_3$ receptor antagonist plus dexamethasone plus an NK-1 receptor antagonist prechemotherapy and dexamethasone plus an NK-1 receptor antagonist post chemotherapy for patients receiving HEC [34–36]. Based on the recent palonosetron studies, palonosetron has been recommended as the preferred 5-HT$_3$ receptor antagonist by multiple international antiemetic guidelines [34–36] for the prevention of acute nausea and vomiting associated with initial and repeat courses of MEC and HEC and for the prevention of delayed nausea and vomiting associated with initial and repeat courses of MEC.

Saito et al. [20] conducted a comparison of palonosetron plus dexamethasone versus granisetron plus dexamethasone for the prevention of CINV in patients receiving HEC.

The palonosetron regimen provided a significantly higher complete response and control of nausea, but neither regimen provided effective control of nausea (no nausea, overall period: 31.9 % palonosetron group; 25.0 % granisetron group) (Table 10.1).

There are no other second-generation 5-HT$_3$ receptor antagonists on the market and there is no information available on other second-generation agents in development.

10.3.3   Aprepitant

Aprepitant is an NK-1 receptor antagonist which blocks the emetic effects of substance-P [4, 5, 37]. When combined with a standard regimen of the corticosteroid dexamethasone and a 5-HT$_3$ receptor antagonist, aprepitant is effective in the prevention of CINV in patients receiving HEC [5, 37]. This regimen is recommended in the guidelines of multiple international groups for the control of CINV in patients receiving HEC [34–36].

Combined data from two large phase III trials of aprepitant plus a first-generation 5-HT$_3$ receptor antagonist and dexamethasone for the prevention of CINV in patients receiving HEC demonstrated an improvement in complete response when aprepitant was added to ondansetron and dexamethasone, but there was no improvement in nausea when the pooled data was analyzed for gender (no nausea, overall period: 46 % for women, aprepitant group, and 38 % for women, control group; 50 % for men, aprepitant group, and 44 % for men, control group) [22] (Table 10.1). Using the same pooled data, a separate analysis [23] showed a statistical but small improvement in no nausea with the use of aprepitant (no nausea, overall period: 48 %, aprepitant group; 42 %, control group) (Table 10.1).

In a similar study involving breast cancer patients receiving cyclophosphamide and doxorubicin or epirubicin, aprepitant was added to ondansetron and dexamethasone for the prevention of CINV. The addition of aprepitant to the 5-HT$_3$ receptor antagonist plus dexamethasone improved the complete response, but there was no improvement in nausea (no nausea, overall period: 33 % aprepitant group; 33 % control group) [37].

Palonosetron and aprepitant have been combined with dexamethasone for the prevention of CINV in a phase II study of 58 patients who received doxorubicin and cyclophosphamide [24]. This three-drug antiemetic regimen was found to be safe and highly effective in preventing emesis and rescue in the acute, delayed, and overall periods, but there was poor control of nausea (no nausea, overall period: 30 %) (Table 10.1).

10.3.4 Netupitant

Netupitant is a new NK-1 receptor antagonist with the structure and a mechanism of action similar to aprepitant, the first agent approved by the FDA in this drug class. Netupitant has a high binding affinity, a long half-life of 90 h, is metabolized by CYP3A4, and is an inhibitor of CYP3A4 [6].

NEPA is an oral fixed-dose combination of netupitant and palonosetron which has recently been employed in phase II and phase III clinical trials for the prevention of CINV in patients receiving MEC and HEC. The clinical trials demonstrated that NEPA (300 mg of netupitant plus 0.50 mg of palonosetron) significantly improved the prevention of CINV compared to the use of palonosetron alone in patients receiving either HEC or MEC. The significant improvement in the delayed period (24–120 h) and the overall period (0–120 h) post chemotherapy was maintained over multiple cycles of chemotherapy. Adverse events were few in number ($\leq$3.5 %) and were mild to moderate in severity. No cardiac adverse events were noted [6].

In an attempt to determine the degree of nausea control with the use of NEPA compared to palonosetron, patients from two randomized, multinational studies who received a single dose of NEPA (netupitant 300 mg plus palonosetron 0.50 mg) or palonosetron and dexamethasone prior to cisplatin or an anthracycline plus cyclophosphamide were evaluated for no significant nausea (<25 mm, 0–100 mm, visual analogue scale). The NEPA group had more patients with no significant nausea and this was most apparent in the delayed nausea phase of the cisplatin patients [6].

On October 10, 2014, NEPA (Akynzeo) was approved by the FDA to treat nausea and vomiting in patients undergoing cancer chemotherapy [6].

10.3.5 Rolapitant

Rolapitant is a high-affinity, highly selective NK-1 receptor antagonist which penetrates the central nervous system following oral administration. It is functionally a competitive antagonist which reverses NK-1 agonist-induced emesis and apomorphine- and cisplatin-induced emesis in animal models. It has a long half-life of approximately 180 h, a high affinity ($K_i = 0.66$ nM) for the NK-1 receptor, and does not induce or inhibit CYP3A4 [7].

A phase I clinical trial in 14 healthy volunteers demonstrated that a – 180 mg rolapitant dose provided ≥90 % NK-1 receptor occupancy in the brain for up to 5 days following a single dose. A phase II randomized, double-blind, active-controlled dose-finding study showed that a 180 mg dose of rolapitant plus granisetron and dexamethasone was safe and effective in the prevention of CINV in patients receiving HEC. CR was significantly improved with rolapitant compared to placebo with all patients receiving ondansetron and dexamethasone.

The 180 mg dose of rolapitant was used in three large phase III clinical trials which demonstrated that rolapitant, granisetron, and dexamethasone significantly improved CR compared to granisetron and dexamethasone alone in patients receiving MEC and HEC. There were no serious adverse events in the two clinical trials, and there were no differences in the number of adverse events in the rolapitant or control arms. No nausea and no significant nausea, secondary endpoints, were significantly ($p < 0.05$) improved in the delayed and overall periods with rolapitant in one (HEC-1) of the two (HEC-1, HEC-2) studies (Table 10.1) [7].

On September 2, 2015, rolapitant (VARUBI) was approved by the FDA to treat nausea and vomiting in patients undergoing cancer chemotherapy.

10.3.6   Dexamethasone

Dexamethasone has been an effective antiemetic in controlling both acute and delayed CINV, and it is essentially the main corticosteroid used as an antiemetic. Concern has been expressed, however, with the potential toxicity of the use of multiple-day dexamethasone to control CINV [38]. Patients receiving dexamethasone for prophylaxis for CINV reported moderate to severe problems with insomnia, hyperglycemia, indigestion, epigastric discomfort, agitation, increased appetite, weight gain, and acne [38]. Dexamethasone might be decreased or eliminated in an antiemetic regime if other agents effective in both the acute and delayed periods are employed.

Dexamethasone added to a 5-HT_3 receptor antagonist improves the control of acute CINV [34–36] and it has been used as a single agent or in combination with other agents in an attempt to control delayed CINV [34–36]. The available studies show that with dexamethasone alone, or combined either with a 5-HT_3 receptor antagonist or metoclopramide in patients receiving cisplatin, the incidence of delayed CINV has been reduced but still remains a significant problem [37]. As an antiemetic, metoclopramide acts as a dopamine antagonist and its action raises the threshold of activity in the chemoreceptor trigger zone and decreases the input from afferent visceral nerves. High doses of metoclopramide have been found to antagonize 5-hydroxytryptamine (5-HT) receptors in the peripheral nervous system in animals.

Celio et al. [25] used palonosetron in combination with a 1-day versus 3 days of dexamethasone to prevent CINV in patients receiving MEC. There was no improvement in complete response (67.5 % versus 71.1) or no nausea (52.1 versus 56.5) over the 5-day overall period. A similar study [39] using palonosetron plus dexamethasone for 1 day versus 3 days for patients receiving MEC showed similar results: no improvement in complete response (53.6 versus 53.7) or in no nausea (47.0 versus 49.7) over the 5-day overall period (Table 10.1).

10.3.7 Olanzapine

Olanzapine is an FDA-approved antipsychotic that blocks multiple neurotransmitters: dopamine at D1, D2, D3, and D4 brain receptors; serotonin at 5-HT_{2a}, 5-HT_{2c}, 5-HT_3, and 5-HT_6 receptors; catecholamines at alpha1 adrenergic receptors; acetylcholine at muscarinic receptors; and histamine at H1 receptors [40, 41]. Common side effects are sedation and weight gain [42, 43], as well as an association with the onset of diabetes mellitus [44]. Significant sedation has not been observed with the doses ($\leq$10 mg/day for 3–5 days) administered for the prevention of CINV [8–10]. Weight gain and the onset of diabetes is observed only when olanzapine is given at higher doses (>10 mg/day) for longer time periods (daily for>3 months) [42–44].

Olanzapine's activity at multiple receptors, particularly at the D2, 5-HT_{2c}, and 5-HT_3 receptors which appear to be involved in nausea and emesis, suggests that it may have significant antiemetic properties.

A phase II trial demonstrated that olanzapine, when combined with a single dose of dexamethasone and a single dose of palonosetron, was very effective in controlling acute and delayed CINV in patients receiving both HEC and MEC [9]. There was excellent control of nausea in 32 patients receiving MEC (no nausea: overall period, 78 %) without the use of multiple days of dexamethasone.

A phase III study showed the addition of olanzapine to the 5-HT_3 receptor antagonist azasetron and dexamethasone improved delayed CINV in patients receiving HEC or MEC [10]. There was a significant improvement in nausea in the olanzapine group compared to the control group for both patients receiving HEC (no nausea, overall period: 70 % versus 28 %) and MEC (no nausea, overall period: 86 % versus 56 %).

A phase III study randomized patients receiving HEC to olanzapine, palonosetron, and dexamethasone (OPD) or aprepitant, palonosetron, and dexamethasone (APD) for the prevention of CINV [27]. The completed response was similar, but no nausea was significantly improved in the OPD group (no nausea, overall period: 69 % versus 38 %). These results were consistent with the previous phase II and phase III studies using olanzapine and suggest that olanzapine is an effective and safe agent for the control of both emesis and nausea (Table 10.1).

10.3.8 Gabapentin

Gabapentin is a gamma-aminobutyric acid analogue which has been used for the treatment of seizures, chronic neuropathic pain, and postherpetic neuralgia [45]. The mechanism of action exerted by gabapentin is unknown. Gabapentin is structurally related to the neurotransmitter GABA, but it does not interact with GABA receptors, is not converted metabolically into GABA or a GABA agonist, and is not an inhibitor of GABA uptake or degradation [45].

Guttuso et al. [46] reported an improvement in CINV in six of nine breast cancer patients when gabapentin was used to prevent nausea. Cruz et al. [28] added gabapentin to ondansetron, dexamethasone, and ranitidine to prevent CINV in patients receiving HEC. The complete response was significantly improved in the patients receiving gabapentin but nausea was not significantly improved (no nausea, overall: 62 % versus 45 %) (Table 10.1).

10.3.9 Cannabinoids

Studies in animal models have suggested that delta-9-tetrahydrocannabinoid (dronabinol) selectively acts on CB1 receptors in specific regions of the dorsal vagal complex to inhibit emesis [47, 48]. There have been few reported studies that have explored this mechanism in patients [29, 49]. Meiri et al. [29] looked at the efficacy of dronabinol versus ondansetron in patients receiving chemotherapy for a wide variety of neoplasms. Dronabinol and ondansetron were similarly effective antiemetic treatments in 61 patients receiving MEC and HEC.

Nabilone is a synthetic cannabinoid, a racemic mixture of isomers, which mimics the main ingredient of cannabis (dronabinol). A recent review of the published English literature on the use of oral nabilone in the treatment of CINV concluded that cannabinoids do not add to benefits of the 5-HT$_3$ receptor antagonists [49]. Additional studies need to be performed to determine the role of this drug class in the prevention or treatment of CINV.

10.3.10 Ginger

Ginger is a herbal supplement which has been used for reducing the severity of motion sickness, pregnancy-induced nausea, and postoperative nausea and vomiting [50]. The mechanism of action by which ginger might exert antiemetic effects is unclear. Animal studies have described enhanced gastrointestinal transport, anti-5-hydroxytryptamine activity, and possible CNS antiemetic effects. Human experiments to determine the mechanism of action show varying results regarding gastric motility and corpus motor response [50].

Pillai et al. [51] added ginger to ondansetron and dexamethasone in children and young adults receiving HEC and reported a reduction in the severity of acute and delayed CINV, but all patients had some nausea in days 1–4 post chemotherapy. Zick et al. [52] reported that ginger provided no additional benefit for reduction of the prevalence or severity of acute or delayed CINV when given with 5-HT$_3$ receptor antagonists and/or aprepitant in 162 cancer patients receiving chemotherapy.

Ryan et al. [53] gave ginger before and after chemotherapy administration to 644 patients receiving a wide variety of chemotherapy regimens and found a reduction in nausea during the first day of chemotherapy. The available studies do not support ginger as an effective agent for the prevention of chemotherapy-induced nausea.

10.4 Discussion

The current data in the literature of multiple large studies suggest that neither the first- nor second-generation 5-HT$_3$ receptor antagonists have been effective in the control of nausea in patients receiving either MEC or HEC, despite the marked improvement in the control of emesis. Similarly, aprepitant, the first NK-1 receptor antagonist to be used clinically for the prevention of CINV, is effective for the control of emesis but not nausea in patients receiving MEC or HEC. This is well documented in multiple large phase III clinical trials.

The new NK-1 receptor antagonists netupitant and rolapitant also do not appear to be effective antinausea agents based on phase III clinical trial data. Rolapitant may have some effect in patients receiving cisplatin HEC. These studies suggest that the serotonin (5HT$_3$) and the substance P (NK-1) receptors may not be the important receptors in the mediation of nausea, despite their important role in chemotherapy-induced emesis.

The recent phase II and phase III studies using olanzapine suggest that this may be an important agent in the control of chemotherapy-induced nausea. Olanzapine is known to affect a wide variety of receptors including dopamine D2, 5-HT$_{2C}$, histaminic, and muscarinic receptors. Any or all of these receptors may be the mediators of chemotherapy-induced nausea.

Preliminary small studies with gabapentin have demonstrated some effectiveness in the control of chemotherapy-induced emesis, but the control of nausea remains to be determined. More studies with the use of cannabinoids need to be performed before it is known whether this class of agents is clinically efficacious in the control of CINV. The studies performed to date do not support the use of ginger as an effective agent in the prevention of CINV.

10.5 Conclusion

It is apparent that the current commonly used antiemetics are not effective for the control of chemotherapy-induced nausea, despite their recent success in the control of emesis. New studies using novel agents and using nausea as the primary endpoint need to be performed. At this point, olanzapine appears to have high potential for the control both emesis and nausea in patients receiving MEC or HEC.

Acknowledgments Supported by the Reich Endowment for the Care of the Whole Patient.

References

1. Bloechl-Daum B, Deuson RR, Panagiotis M et al (2006) Delayed nausea and vomiting continue to reduce patients' quality of life after highly and moderately emetogenic chemotherapy despite antiemetic treatment. J Clin Oncol 24:4472–4478
2. Navari RM (2009) Pharmacological management of chemotherapy-induced nausea and vomiting: focus on recent developments. Drugs 69:515–533
3. Navari RM (2010) Palonosetron for the prevention of chemotherapy-induced nausea and vomiting in patients with cancer. Future Oncol 6:1073–1084
4. Curran MP, Robinson DM (2009) Aprepitant: a review of its use in the prevention of nausea and vomiting. Drugs 69:1853–1858
5. Sankhala KK, Pandya DM, Sarantopoulos J et al (2009) Prevention of chemotherapy induced nausea and vomiting: a focus on aprepitant. Expert Opin Drug Metab Toxicol 12:1607–1614
6. Navari RM (2015) Profile of netupitant/palonosetron fixed dose combination (NEPA) and its potential in the treatment of chemotherapy-induced nausea and vomiting (CINV. Drug Des Dev Ther 9:155–161
7. Navari RM (2015) Rolapitant for the treatment of chemotherapy induced nausea and vomiting. Expert Rev Anticancer Ther 15:1127–1133
8. Navari RM, Einhorn LH, Loehrer PJ et al (2005) A phase II trial of olanzapine for the prevention of chemotherapy-induced nausea and vomiting. Support Care Cancer 13:529–534
9. Navari RM, Einhorn LH, Loehrer PJ et al (2007) A phase II trial of olanzapine, dexamethasone, and palonosetron for the prevention of chemotherapy-induced nausea and vomiting. Support Care Cancer 15:1285–1291
10. Tan L, Liu J, Liu X et al (2009) Clinical research of olanzapine for the prevention of chemotherapy-induced nausea and vomiting. J Exp Clin Cancer Res 28:1–7
11. Stern RM, Koch KL, Andrews PLR (2011) Nausea: mechanisms and management. Oxford University Press, New York
12. Simpson K, Spencer CM, McClellan KJ (2000) Tropisetron: an update of its use in the prevention of chemotherapy-induced nausea and vomiting. Drugs 59:1297–1315
13. Kimura E, Niimi E, Wantabe A et al (1996) Study on the clinical effect of a continuous intravenous infusion of azasetron against nausea and vomiting induced by anticancer drugs including CDDP. Gan To Kagaku Ryoho 23:477–481
14. Taguchi T, Tsukamoto F, Watanabe T et al (1999) Usefulness of ramosetron hydrochloride on nausea and vomiting in CMF or CEF therapy for breast cancer. Gan To Kagaku Ryoho 26:1163–1170
15. Dolasetron drug alert. WHO Drug Information, 40, No. 3 (2006)
16. U.S. Food and Drug Information. FDA drug safety communication: abnormal heart rhythms associated with use of Anzemet (dolasetron mesylate). Available from URL: http://www.fda.gov/Drugs.DrugSafety/usm237081.htm. Accessed 27 Dec 2010
17. Roila F, Warr D, Clark-Snow R et al (2005) Delayed emesis: moderately emetogenic chemotherapy. Support Care Cancer 13(2):104–108
18. Geling O, Eichler H (2005) Should 5-Hydroxytryptamine-3 receptor antagonists be administered beyond 24 hours after chemotherapy to prevent delayed emesis? Systematic re-evaluation of clinical evidence and drug cost implications. J Clin Oncol 23:1289–1294
19. Hickok JT, Roscoe JA, Morrow GR et al (2005) 5-HT$_3$ receptor antagonists versus prochlorperazine for control of delayed nausea caused by doxorubicin: a URCC CCOP randomized controlled trial. Lancet Oncol 6:765–772
20. Saito M, Aogi K, Sekine I et al (2009) Palonosetron plus dexamethasone versus granisetron plus dexamethasone for the prevention of nausea and vomiting during chemotherapy: a double-blind, double dummy, randomized, comparative phase III trial. Lancet Oncol 10:115–124
21. Warr DG, Hesketh PJ, Gralla RJ et al (2005) Efficacy and tolerability of aprepitant for the prevention of chemotherapy-induced nausea and vomiting in patients with breast cancer after moderately emetogenic chemotherapy. J Clin Oncol 23:2822–2830

22. Hesketh PJ, Grunberg SM, Herrstedt J et al (2006) Combined data from two phase III trials of the NK-1 antagonist aprepitant plus a 5HT$_3$ antagonist and a corticosteroid for prevention of chemotherapy-induced nausea and vomiting: effect of gender on treatment response. Support Care Cancer 14:354–360

23. Warr DG, Grunberg SM, Gralla RJ et al (2005) The oral NK1 antagonist aprepitant for the prevention of acute and delayed chemotherapy-induced nausea and vomiting: pooled data from two randomized, double-blind, placebo controlled trials. Eur J Cancer 41:1278–1285

24. Grote T, Hajdenberg Cartnell A et al (2006) Combination therapy for chemotherapy-induced nausea and vomiting in patients receiving moderately emetogenic chemotherapy: palonosetron, dexamethasone, and aprepitant. J Support Oncol 4:408

25. Celio L, Frustaci S, Denaro A et al (2011) Palonosetron in combination with 1-day versus 3-day dexamethasone for prevention of nausea and vomiting following moderately emetogenic chemotherapy: a randomized, multi-center, phase III trial. Support Care Cancer 19:1217–1225

26. Aapro MS, Grunberg SM, Manikhas GM et al (2006) A phase III, double blind, randomized trial of palonosetron compared with ondansetron in preventing chemotherapy-induced nausea and vomiting following highly emetogenic chemotherapy. Ann Oncol 17:1441–1449

27. Navari RM, Gray SE, Kerr AC (2011) Olanzapine versus aprepitant for the control of chemotherapy-induced nausea and vomiting: a randomized phase III trial. J Support Oncol (in press)

28. Cruz FM, de Iracema Gomes Cubero D, Taranto P (2011) Gabapentin for the prevention of chemotherapy-induced nausea and vomiting: a pilot study. Support Care Cancer (in press)

29. Meiri E, Jhangiani H, Vredenburgh JJ et al (2007) Efficacy of dronabinol alone and in combination with ondansetron versus ondansetron alone for delayed chemotherapy-induced nausea and vomiting. Curr Med Res Opin 23:533–543

30. Eisenberg P, MacKintosh FR, Ritch P et al (2004) Efficacy, safety, and pharmacokinetics of palonosetron in patients receiving highly emetogenic, cisplatin-based chemotherapy: a dose-ranging, clinical study. Ann Oncol 15:330–337

31. Rojas C, Thomas AG, Alt J et al (2010) Palonosetron triggers 5-HT$_3$ receptor internalization and causes prolonged inhibition of receptor function. J Pharmacol 626:193–199

32. Eisenberg P, Figueroa-Vadillo J, Zamora R et al (2003) Improved prevention of moderately emetogenic chemotherapy-induced nausea and vomiting with palonosetron, a pharmacologically novel 5HT3 receptor antagonist: results of a phase III, single dose trial versus dolasetron. Cancer 98:2473–2482

33. Gralla R, Lichinitser M, Van der Vegt S et al (2003) Palonosetron improves prevention of chemotherapy-induced nausea and vomiting following moderately emetogenic chemotherapy: results of a double-blind randomized phase II trial comparing single dose of palonosetron with ondansetron. Ann Oncol 14:1570–1577

34. Basch E, Prestrud AA, Hesketh PJ et al (2011) Antiemetic American Society Clinical Oncology clinical practice guideline update. J Clin Oncol 29:4189–4198

35. NCCN National Comprehensive Cancer Network (2015) Antiemesis: Clinical Practice Guidelines in Oncology. v 1. www.nccn.org

36. Roila F, Herrstedt J, Aapro M et al (2010) Guideline update for MASCC and ESMO in the prevention of chemotherapy- and radiotherapy-induced nausea and vomiting: results of the Perugia consensus conference. Ann Oncol 21(Suppl 5):232–243

37. Navari RM (2003) Pathogenesis-based treatment of chemotherapy-induced nausea and vomiting: two new agents. J Support Oncol 1:89–103

38. Vardy J, Chiew KS, Gallica J et al (1999) Side effects associated with the use of dexamethasone for prophylaxis of delayed emesis after moderately emetogenic chemotherapy. Br J Cancer 94:1011–1015

39. Aapro M, Fabi A, Nole F et al (2010) Double-blind, randomized, controlled study of the efficacy and tolerability of palonosetron plus dexamethasone for 1 day with or without dexamethasone on days 2 and 3 in the prevention of nausea and vomiting induced by moderately emetogenic chemotherapy. Ann Oncol 21:1083–1088

40. Bymaster FP, Calligaro D, Falcone J et al (1996) Radioreceptor binding profile of the atypical antipsychotic olanzapine. Neuropsychopharmacology 14:87–96
41. Bymaster FP, Falcone JF, Bauzon D et al (2001) Potent antagonism of 5HT3 and 5HT6 receptors by olanzapine. Eur J Pharmacol 430:341–349
42. Allison DB, Casey DE (2001) Antipsychotic-associated weight gain: a review of the literature. J Clin Psychiatry 62:22–31
43. Hale AS (1997) Olanzapine. Br J Hosp Med 58:443–445
44. Goldstein LE, Sporn J, Brown S et al (1999) New-onset diabetes mellitus and diabetic ketoacidosis associated with olanzapine treatment. Psychosomatics 40:438–443
45. Irving G, Jensen M, Cramer M et al (2009) Efficacy and tolerability of gastric-retentive gabapentin for the treatment of post-herpetic neuralgia: results of a double-blind, randomized, placebo-controlled clinical trial. Clin J Pain 25(3):185–192
46. Guttuso T, Roscoe J, Griggs J (2003) Effect of gabapentin on nausea induced by chemotherapy in patients with breast cancer. Lancet 361:1703–1705
47. Van Sickle MD, Oland LD, Mackie K et al (2003) Delta9-tetrahydrocannabinol selectively acts on CB1 receptors in specific regions of dorsal vagal complex to inhibit emesis in ferrets. Am J Physiol Gastrointest Liver Physiol 285:G566–G576
48. Darmani NA (2001) Delta-9-tetrahydrocannabinol differentially suppresses cisplatin-induced emesis and indices of motor function via cannabinoid CB1 receptors in the least shrew. Pharmacol Biochem Behav 69:239–249
49. Davis MP (2008) Oral nabilone capsules in the treatment of chemotherapy-induced nausea and vomiting and pain. Expert Opin Investig Drugs 17(1):85–95
50. Mills S, Bone K (2000) Principles and practice of phytotherapy. Churchill Livingstone, Oxford
51. Pillai AK, Sharma KK, Gupta YK, Bakhshi S (2011) Anti-emetic effect of ginger powder versus placebo as an add-on therapy in children and young adults receiving high emetogenic chemotherapy. Pediatr Blood Cancer 56:234–238
52. Zick SM, Ruffin MT, Normolle DP et al (2009) Phase II trial of encapsulated ginger as a treatment for chemotherapy-induced nausea and vomiting. Support Care Cancer 17:563–572
53. Ryan JL, Heckler C, Dakhil SR et al (2009) Ginger for chemotherapy-related nausea in cancer patients: a URCC CCOP randomized, double-blind, placebo-controlled clinical trial of 644 cancer patients. J Clin Oncol 27(15s):abstract 9511

Chapter 11
Conclusions

Rudolph M. Navari

The first-generation $5\text{-}HT_3$ receptor antagonists (dolasetron, granisetron, ondansetron, tropisetron, ramosetron, and azasetron) have significant and similar efficacy in the prevention of acute CINV for patients receiving moderately emetogenic chemotherapy (MEC) and highly emetogenic chemotherapy (HEC). These agents do not appear to have significant efficacy in the prevention of delayed CINV, and these agents compete primarily on an economic basis.

The second-generation $5\text{-}HT_3$ receptor antagonist palonosetron improves the complete response rate of acute and delayed emesis in patients receiving MEC and HEC. The current data in the literature of multiple large studies suggest that neither the first- nor the second-generation $5\text{-}HT_3$ receptor antagonists have been effective in the control of nausea in patients receiving either MEC or HEC, despite the marked improvement in the control of emesis.

The NK_1 receptor antagonists aprepitant, netupitant, and rolapitant significantly improve the control of acute and delayed CINV when added to a $5\text{-}HT_3$ receptor antagonist and dexamethasone for patients receiving HEC and MEC. The NK_1 receptor antagonists do not appear to be effective as antinausea agents.

Recently completed phase II and phase III clinical trials have demonstrated that the use of olanzapine in combination with a $5\text{-}HT_3$ receptor antagonist and dexamethasone is safe and effective in the prevention of emesis and nausea in patients receiving MEC and HEC.

Olanzapine appears to be an important agent in the control of chemotherapy-induced nausea. Olanzapine is known to affect a wide variety of receptors, including

R.M. Navari, MD, PhD, FACP
Cancer Care Program, Central and South America, World Health Organization,
Atlanta, USA

Student Outreach Clinic, Indiana University School of Medicine South Bend,
South Bend, IN, USA
e-mail: rmnavari@gmail.com

© Springer International Publishing Switzerland 2016
R.M. Navari (ed.), *Management of Chemotherapy-Induced Nausea
and Vomiting: New Agents and New Uses of Current Agents*,
DOI 10.1007/978-3-319-27016-6_11

dopamine D2, $5\text{-}HT_{2C}$, $5\text{-}HT_3$, and histaminic and muscarinic receptors. Any or all of these receptors may be the mediators of chemotherapy-induced nausea.

A recent randomized phase III clinical trial demonstrated that olanzapine also appears to be an effective agent in the treatment of chemotherapy-induced breakthrough emesis and nausea.

Preliminary small studies with gabapentin have demonstrated some effectiveness in the control of chemotherapy-induced emesis, but the control of nausea remains to be determined. The studies on the use of cannabinoids and ginger do not support the use of these agents as effective in the prevention of CINV.

Clinicians and other healthcare professionals who are involved in administering chemotherapy should be aware that studies have strongly suggested that patients experience more acute and delayed CINV than is perceived by practitioners, and patients often do not receive adequate prophylaxis. A number of international organizations have published extensive guidelines on the use of prophylactic antiemetic regimens as well as directives on the management of patients with breakthrough, refractory, and anticipatory CINV.

Oncology practitioners are encouraged to use the evidence-based guidelines for the prevention of CINV.

Palonosetron, aprepitant, netupitant, rolapitant, and olanzapine have not been studied extensively in multi-day chemotherapy, bone marrow transplantation, or radiotherapy-induced nausea and vomiting. Future studies may address whether these agents would be effective in patients who experience nausea and vomiting during these clinical settings. Future studies may determine not only how these agents should be used and what combinations of new and older agents will be the most beneficial for patients but may also provide new information on the mechanism of CINV.

Chapter 12
Future Directions

Rudolph M. Navari

The various international clinical guidelines have consistently recommended the use of the combination of the antiemetic agents discussed in this text for the prevention of CINV. It is anticipated that the 5-HT$_3$ receptor antagonists will continue to be used extensively in the preventative regimens due to their high efficacy in the prevention of emesis. The choice of whether to use ondansetron, granisetron, or palonosetron will be dependent on the issues of cost and efficacy. Palonosetron is the recommended agent of this class by the international guidelines based on efficacy, but its cost may be an issue for some institutions compared to the generic availability of ondansetron and granisetron. At this time, there do not appear to be other 5-HT$_3$ receptor antagonists in development for commercial use.

Even though the mechanism of dexamethasone as an antiemetic is unknown, it appears to be very effective for the prevention of acute and delayed CINV. There have been no serious toxicities reported with 1–4-day uses in the various clinical trials. Some recent trials have suggested that 1 day of dexamethasone pre-chemotherapy may be equivalent in efficacy to 3 days. Future trials may further explore this issue.

At present, there are no definitive clinical trials reporting a comparison of the efficacy and safety of the various NK$_1$ receptor antagonists (aprepitant, fosaprepitant, netupitant, rolapitant). One of the NEPA clinical trials involving patients receiving highly emetogenic chemotherapy (HEC) included a comparative arm consisting of oral aprepitant plus intravenous ondansetron. All patients in all arms received standard doses of dexamethasone. Based on the data reported in this NEPA

R.M. Navari, MD, PhD, FACP
Cancer Care Program, Central and South America, World Health Organization, Atlanta, USA

Student Outreach Clinic, Indiana University School of Medicine South Bend, South Bend, IN, USA
e-mail: rmnavari@gmail.com

© Springer International Publishing Switzerland 2016
R.M. Navari (ed.), *Management of Chemotherapy-Induced Nausea and Vomiting: New Agents and New Uses of Current Agents*,
DOI 10.1007/978-3-319-27016-6_12

clinical trial, there appeared to be no significant differences in the prevention of CINV between NEPA and the aprepitant and ondansetron combination. A formal statistical comparison of the NEPA and aprepitant/ondansetron arms was not reported.

The NEPA clinical trials and the rolapitant clinical trials were designed to compare each of the new NK_1 receptor antagonists plus a $5\text{-}HT_3$ receptor antagonist and dexamethasone to a $5\text{-}HT_3$ receptor antagonist and dexamethasone alone. The study design was similar to the clinical trial which led to the approval of the first NK_1 aprepitant in 2003. The studies were not designed to compare the new NK_1 receptor antagonists to aprepitant, the commercially available NK_1, at the time of the studies. It is not known whether this was a decision made by the study sponsor(s) or by a regulatory agency. As a result, there is currently little or no clinical trial comparison of efficacy information available for practicing oncologists and patients to base their choice of available NK_1s.

The major clinical studies of the NK_1 receptor antagonists have been performed with oral agents, with fosaprepitant being the only commercially available intravenous NK_1 agent. The clinical importance of the availability of an intravenous form of a specific NK_1 remains to be determined. In addition, it is important to note that netupitant is not available as a single agent; it is only commercially available in combination with palonosetron.

Based on the available clinical trial data, the NK_1 receptor antagonists have significantly improved the prevention of acute and delayed emesis in patients receiving MEC or HEC. There is little evidence, however, that these agents are effective in controlling nausea. Recent reviews have concluded that aprepitant has little effect on the prevention of chemotherapy-induced nausea. In a subgroup analysis of patients receiving cisplatin or an anthracycline plus cyclophosphamide, data from two clinical trials demonstrated that NEPA may have improved no significant nausea (a secondary endpoint) compared to palonosetron. The rolapitant clinical trials showed no improvement in the control of nausea in the patients receiving MEC and improvement in the control of nausea in one of the two trials in patients receiving HEC.

At present, there do not appear to be data which differentiate the three NK_1 receptor antagonists in terms of efficacy and/or safety, and until comparative studies are performed, the three agents appear to be similar for the prevention of CINV. The determining factors in the choice of the NK_1 receptor antagonists will be cost and the preference for the use of either an oral or an intravenous agent. Fosaprepitant is the only intravenous agent available in 2015. It is unknown whether intravenous forms of netupitant will be available in the near future. In May 2015, the manufacturer of rolapitant announced the successful completion of a rolapitant bioequivalence study. The results of the study indicated that the exposure for a 166.5 mg dose of intravenous rolapitant was similar to the exposure of a 180 mg dose of oral rolapitant. It is anticipated that intravenous rolapitant will be available in 2016.

Other possible considerations for the choice of an NK_1 receptor antagonist by oncologists will be the choice of which $5\text{-}HT_3$ receptor antagonist to use with the

NK$_1$ receptor antagonists. At present, netupitant is only available for use in combination with palonosetron.

Although there appear to be other NK$_1$ receptor antagonists in development, there do not appear to be any which are pending regulatory approval in the near future.

There have been a number of phase III clinical trials demonstrating the benefit of olanzapine for the prevention of chemotherapy-induced nausea and emesis. The efficacy of olanzapine for decreasing nausea is in contrast to the control of nausea in clinical trials of the NK$_1$ receptor antagonists. Nausea has not been significantly improved by the use of fosaprepitant (aprepitant) in two phase III studies of patients receiving cisplatin and in two phase III studies of patients receiving an anthracycline and cyclophosphamide chemotherapy regimen. The recent clinical trials used by the FDA for the approval of netupitant and rolapitant did not demonstrate effective control of nausea. Two reviews on the prevention of chemotherapy-induced nausea concluded that NK$_1$ receptor antagonists are not effective in controlling nausea.

The data from the currently reported clinical trials support NCCN guidelines which list the olanzapine, palonosetron, and dexamethasone regimen as an optional first-line therapy for the prevention of CINV in patients receiving HEC.

There are economic benefits of olanzapine. Four days of generic oral olanzapine at 10 mg/day, the dose used in this study and previous prophylactic studies, is approximately $3.00 which is significantly lower than the cost of 1 day of intravenous fosaprepitant at 150 mg (approximate wholesale acquisition cost, $257.00).

Olanzapine appeared to be well tolerated in the various clinical trials. In the randomized, double-blind clinical trial of patients receiving HEC, patients who received olanzapine had more drowsiness on day 2 compared to baseline, but this was resolved by day 3 despite continued oral olanzapine on days 3 and 4, suggesting that patients adapted to the olanzapine. Due to the temporary drowsiness seen in this trial and reports of temporary drowsiness in some patients, more detailed data on drowsiness ratings should be obtained in future trials. To conclude, there is definitive clinical trial convincing evidence that olanzapine does decrease nausea and vomiting associated with chemotherapy. Future investigations may include exploring the efficacy of olanzapine as an oral agent for the treatment of chronic nausea, unrelated to chemotherapy, as well as for clinical situations such as multi-day chemotherapy or high-dose chemotherapy and stem cell transplantation.